M000206457

DR. ZEEV GILKIS

RUNNING
BACK
IN TIME

• • • • • • • • • • • • • • • • • • •

*Discovering the Formula to Beat
the Aging Process and Get Younger*

Producer & International Distributor
eBookPro Publishing
www.ebook-pro.com

Running Back In Time
Dr. Zeev Gilkis

Illustrations by Omri Gilkis

Contact: zeev.gilkis@yahoo.com
ISBN: 9789655751598

RUNNING
BACK
IN TIME

•••••••••••••••••••••••

*Discovering the Formula to Beat
the Aging Process and Get Younger*

DR. ZEEV GILKIS

Contents

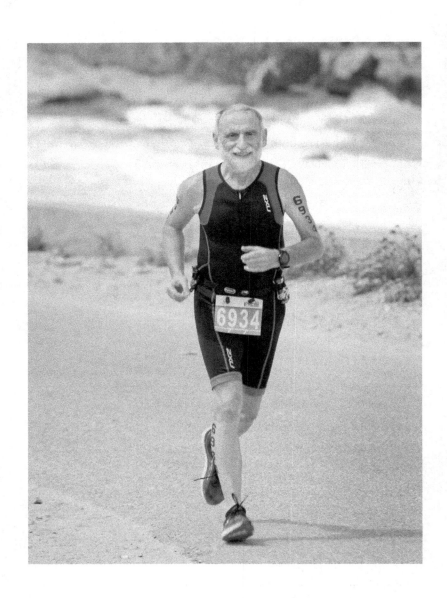

CHAPTER 1
···············
An Unusual Birthday Present

March 1st 2019. My 68th birthday!

I'm going to "write" the next pages of the book of my life.

I mean – I want to create the reality, and then to write about it.

Is the SKY the limit?!

Well, it depends what you mean by this question.

When I was five, I asked my parents whether the sky has a "ceiling." And, if there is a "roof" over the sky, what's above it?

When I was running 1.5 kilometers once a week, 3 kilometers was my "sky"… After some training I became a competitive 10K runner.

So, everything is relative.

My answer to this question is in Chapter 18; "Mind Over Matter."

I'm beginning my new memoir.

Although in the coming two years I'll be closing my 7th decade, I still have a lot of plans and a lot of expectations for the coming years.

Shimon Peres the ninth President of Israel, once said at the age of 91: *"The bigger the dreams and aspirations a person has, the younger he is!"*

I have many plans and dreams, but the biggest challenge I'm setting for myself for the near future, is to run my first marathon on my 70th birthday.

It definitely may seem like a fantasy, and maybe it is.

I loved Paulo Coelho's "The Pilgrimage," even more than "The Alchemist." In this book he beautifully demonstrates that the journey toward a goal is much more important than achieving the goal!

I can't know now whether or not I'll achieve my goal, but I definitely intend to enjoy the journey!

This specific journey is only a fraction of the big JOURNEY OF LIFE. So, let's enjoy LIFE!

You, the reader, will be my companion on this challenging path and I promise to share everything with you; the good and the bad, the ups and the downs, the joy and the disappointments.
I'm sure we both will learn from it. Are you ready?!

You may be asking: "Why do you have to run a marathon at the age of 70??"

This is definitely a good question.

I'll divide the answer into two parts:

I strongly believe in the benefits of sports activities:

In addition to strengthening the immune system, and contributing greatly to the functioning and performance of the cardiovascular and cardio-respiratory systems, sports activities protect our brain from neuro-degenerative diseases and mental illnesses, improve our self-esteem and overall satisfaction, and help us to establish a good understanding of and communication with our bodies.

All in all, **the best investment that we can make is in our own health,** in order to improve our quality of life and to secure our future – so that we may grow old in a state of good health, filled with vitality.

Nowadays, increasing numbers of researchers are in agreement that even more than intellectual activity physical activity contributes not only to physical health, but also to mental health.

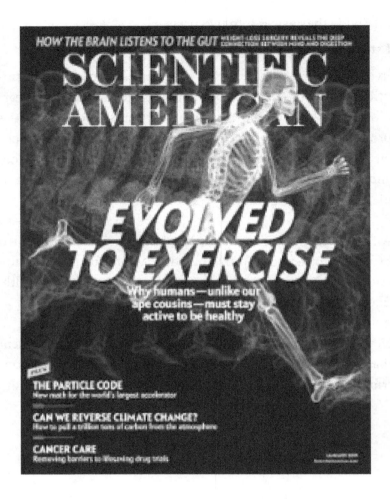

Some studies have found evidence of a high correlation between neurogenesis (the birth of new neurons produced by neural stem cells) in the hippocampus portion of the human brain and physical activity.

The hippocampus is closely linked with the brain's processing of memory.

Therefore, running improves the functioning of our memory!

The second part of the answer is that setting such goals helps me to motivate myself to be physically active.

Obviously, intellectually, I fully understand the life-changing importance of sport activity.

I believe that you do too.

As do many others. But very few actually implement this understanding in their daily lives.

The setting of physically challenging goals definitely serves as a good tool for motivating ourselves. Tracking our progress in reaching these goals acts synergistically with goal setting to strengthen our motivation even more.

I set long-term goals, interim goals and tactical, short-term goals.

To run a marathon on my 70th birthday is a strategic long-term goal.

It is quite ambitious, almost a "mission impossible" from my current perspective.

Maybe this is one of the reasons, why I am so attracted to setting such a goal.

Another, additional, reason is my personal curiosity – can I actually achieve such a goal?! Can I do this physically?! How will it feel?!

Are there limits to achieving the goals we set?!

A few months ago I was diagnosed with a partial tear in the patellar tendon in my knee, and was told to stop running.

This was my second serious injury (not counting the minor

ones), following a double tear in the meniscus, which was operated on in the summer of 2017.

In that operation I lost half of the medial meniscus and was also told for the first time, to stop running.

But I couldn't. In the CAGE Test, I discovered that I'm addicted...

CAGE serves mainly to test whether one is addicted to alcohol, but not only alcohol.

The name CAGE is an acronym of the test's four questions, as follows:

1. Have you ever felt you needed to Cut down on your drinking?
2. Have people Annoyed you by criticizing your drinking?
3. Have you ever felt Guilty about drinking?
4. Have you ever felt you needed a drink first thing in the morning (Eye-opener) to steady your nerves or to get rid of a hangover?

I enjoy a glass of red wine with dinner, usually Cabernet Sauvignon or Pinot Noir. At Saturday morning family breakfasts and on other special occasions, I may have a single malt whisky. I especially like the 12 year old Balvenie.

If you reply positively to two out of the four questions above, then you are considered an alcoholic, at least to a certain extent.

I wish to make it clear – although I do enjoy good wine or whisky from time to time, I am not an alcoholic!

During my recent stay in India, I didn't even smell alcohol for three weeks. There was no opportunity... the drinks there were mainly ginger water and chai masala. Nevertheless, I really did not miss having access to alcohol.

I have never started a morning with a drink and I really don't feel guilty when indulging in this small pleasure. In regard to "A," yes, it's true that sometimes my family annoys me when alluding to my drinking which has become something of a family joke.

So, what am I addicted to?!

When I applied the same test to my running, the result was CAGE 4 meaning that I could relate to four out of the four questions!

Now I was also being told to stop surfing as well, because the condition I was suffering, (the partial patellar tendon tear) is known as "the jumper's knee," and typically occurs among people who jump, and during surfing, when you "catch a wave," you have to "pop-up" – which means performing a very quick and physically demanding jump.

I have been exercising self-discipline, and for the last two months I haven't run at all.

Nor have I surfed.

But I'm addicted. I can't live without running.

So, I decided to gradually start running again but this time in a very limited manner.

I began initially with very short runs: the first one was a 1.5km run, the second a 2km run, and then I ran for 3kms – no pain!

I extended the runs to twice – and then three times a week, running between 3 and 5 kilometers, but no more than 5.

At the same time, I continued with physiotherapy while exercising a lot at home.

I believe that strengthening the muscles and especially the core muscles, will help to better spread the load out over the knees and that this will hopefully help me to avoid additional injuries.

Now I'm running 5kms once a week, taking a two-day break from running afterward (but still swimming or biking) and the other two weekly runs are shorter (just 3-4 kms).

One of the shorter runs includes interval training.

The key principle of interval running is alternating high-intensity running with a period of recovery. For example, I might run hard for a minute or two, followed by an easier two-minute recovery period, in which I jog until my heart beat rate slows down.

I then repeat this cycle several times.

The benefit of interval running is that it improves running efficiency increasing your ability to maintain higher speeds for longer. I love it!

Indeed, my running time is improving, from 7 minutes a kilometer to around 5:30/km.

My interim goals are quite ambitious too; running half marathons. Obviously not now. The first one (the first in my life) will take place at the beginning of November, eight months from the time of this writing.

The plan is to increase my running distances very gradually, reaching 10 kilometers in June.

Then a faster progress, adding one kilometer every 3 to 4 weeks, reaching a maximal range of 17 to 18 kilometers in October.

Hopefully, this will provide me with a sufficient base from which to make the extra 3-4km effort needed to run the 21.1km half marathon in November.

All these are plans.

To realize them I'll have to do a lot of work, on a daily basis; outdoors and at home – these are the short-term goals.

Below is a sample of my runs during the last six weeks

DATE	DIST	TIME	PACE	AHR	MHR	SPM	SL
18-01-19	3.81	21:03	5:32	156	184	165	1.10
21-01-19	3.57	21:17	5:58	150	169	164	1.02
25-01-19	3.81	22:19	5:51	153	171	163	1.05
28-01-19	5.09	27:52	5:29	158	177	170	1.07
30-01-19	3.85	22:51	5:56	149	169	158	1.07
01-02-19	4.01	21:38	5:24	155	174	170	1.09
03-02-19	5.17	28:28	5:30	154	173	165	1.10
05-02-19	4.01	22:01	5:29	153	174	163	1.12
08-02-19	5.38	30:34	5:41	157	171	163	1.08
13-02-19	5.42	31:42	5:51	154	169	160	1.07
19-02-19	5.45	31:32	5:47	154	173	163	1.06
21-02-19	4.43	24:30	5:32	155	172	165	1.10
24-02-19	5.52	30:04	5:27	159	175	165	1.11
28-02-19	4.46	24:20	5:28	143	168	168	1.09

DIST - the run distance in kilometers
TIME - the overall time of the run
PACE - how many minutes it takes me to run 1km
AHR - average heart rate
MHR - maximum heart rate
SPM - steps per minute
SL - stride length in meters

The pace, below 6min/km is good enough, but you have to consider that these are 4-5km runs of up to a half hour each, while the half-marathon (21.1km) will most probably take me at least 2.5 hours, because I'll have to run at a much slower pace (I am assuming at 7min/km, or maybe even a bit slower).

The good news is, that the AHR is always below 160 – my lactic threshold (LT).

The lactate threshold is the maximum exercise intensity (as measured by the heartbeat rate), before which the blood concentration of lactic acid begins to exponentially increase.

In other words, an intensity, that an athlete can maintain for an extended period of time with little or no increase of lactate in the blood.

When exercising at or below the LT, any lactate produced by the muscles is removed by the body without it building up.

Regular endurance exercise leads to adaptations in skeletal muscle which prevent lactate levels from rising.

The maximum heart rate is usually below 175 and that's fine too.

Also, the HR returns to normal quite fast; to 120 after two minutes and to around 100 after 5 minutes.

The stride length of around 110cms is quite good, even a bit too extended. A stride that is too long is dangerous and running with long strides can make one more prone to injuries.

I used to run with much shorter strides, less than a meter, but at a much higher cadence, usually at around 170.

I'll have to work on these two key parameters and find the optimal balance.

The goals are set and now we can begin the journey!

Setting goals leaves no room for doubt – I know where I'm heading.

Also, by now my body and my mind know as well.

And they seem to be terrified.

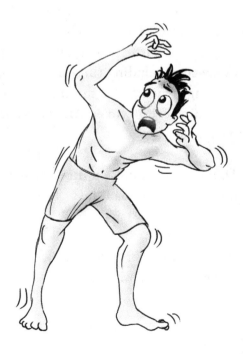

I ended my second book "The Secret of Life, a memoir of getting younger," with a promise, that despite the second injury, **I'll be back on track!**

The synopsis of "my story" until then is:

a mathematician, with a PhD in Artificial Intelligence, and a long career in hi-tech, bio-tech and venture capital who successfully completed a battle with advanced stage colorectal cancer (stage 3 out of 4).

Since overcoming cancer I have gradually increased my involvement in sport activities with an inflection point occurring at age 66, when I for the first time, competed in a triathlon.

Although I began involvement in sports only in my sixties, which might be considered a bit late in life, my level of involvement is relatively high; I participate in one activity or another at least 5 times a week: including running, biking, swimming and basic exercising. During the summer this may include surfing, and I go skiing every winter. And occasionally I go on a scuba diving trip.

Now, you will be my companion on this two-year journey, although you might be able to read the story of these two years in two days, if you wish.

But it's my job to construct the story, to work hard with my "bare hands." Or maybe with my legs.

So far, the maximum distance I have run is a 15km run and not that many times; twice in January 2018 and three times in July 2018, all in all, five times. My best time was 88 minutes which included an unpleasant pain in my left foot.

In July 2018 when I overdid it (running 15kms-10kms-15kms in one week), I got the partial tear in the patellar tendon.

Now I intend to be more careful, making it a point to take longer breaks after the longer runs so as to allow the body to heal from the inevitable micro-tears and micro-trauma.

You will be my buddy, as I tell you about all of the ups and downs, and I can assure you, from my personal experience, there are always "downs" to deal with…

That's why mental strength is so crucial on such a long and challenging path.

I have found that the Transcendental Meditation that I have practiced for over 40 years is usually very helpful in such situations.

Everything (like the decision to run the marathon) begins in the mind! And the mind controls your entire path in life …

My decision to run a marathon, at this stage expressed only to myself and only through the pages of this memoir, is the basis on which I set my expectations for myself.

Consequently, my body is beginning to understand what my personal expectations are …

It is I who sets the stage…

CHAPTER 2
••••••••••••••
The White Dream, Skiing in Poland

As I write these words, I am concluding a 10-day ski vacation in Szklarska Poręba, a small ski town in the Karkonosze Mountains in the Sudetes in southwestern Poland, along the border with the Czech Republic.

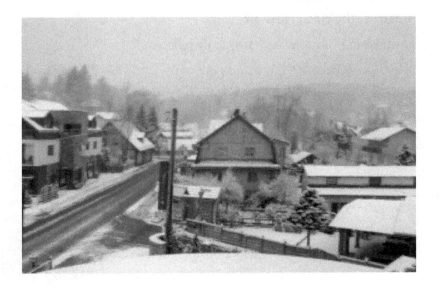

I usually go at the beginning of March. That is the end of the season, so there are less people, shorter lines, and the skiing conditions are usually still quite good.

There is a saying: "People don't stop because they get older, they get older, because they stop, or slow down."

I do not intend to slow down…

Each sport discipline is unique, but diversifying and switching from one discipline to another makes it more interesting, never becoming boring.

There is also a synergy, especially on the level of mind and body.

I love skiing not only because of the activity itself, but also because of what I can view around me.

I love the white landscapes, the trees covered with a silky-white dressing, the clean clear air.

And when it is snowing, it is really beautiful!

Maybe also because it reminds me of my childhood. Although when I was a young boy in Poland I wasn't a skier, but I grew up with white winters every year.

And of course I love the speed.

As with the other sports activities I began a bit late, at the age of 63.

It began with a beautiful photo my cousin Jurek sent me from his cross-country ski with his son, when everything around them was white.

So, the next year I came for a week of cross-country skiing.

I also tried some downhill skiing, but had trouble stopping myself, I fell a few times and gave up.

But the next year I came again. This time, Dorota, the instructor, taught me stopping and I gained some confidence.

Since then I ski at least a week each year. My daily session comprises one hour with Tomek, an excellent instructor, and another 2 to 3 hours on my own.

Each year there is further progress and more joy and satisfaction.

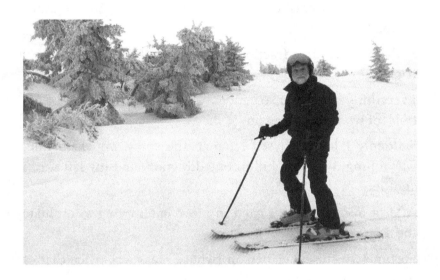

This year the skiing conditions were ideal, and occasional sprinklings of snow added to the overall experience.

There were not many people, especially in the early morning hours, when I would begin.

The first three days passed smoothly and I really enjoyed myself.

But on the fourth day…

I was skiing at a moderate speed; like maybe 30 kms/hour when a large group of beginners, following their instructor, started crossing the hill in front of me from right to left.

There were several 2 to 3 meter "windows" or spaces, between them, and my only option was to get through one of those windows.

I picked one, but unfortunately the person I had been planning to pass behind suddenly stopped! Not being able to avoid him I unfortunately crashed into him with all of my 60 kilograms of weight.

It all happened in a fraction of a second, but it was extremely frightening.

Everything happened so suddenly and so fast, I couldn't keep track of what was going on.

Suddenly I found myself lying in the snow, my ski helmet was rolling down the hill in one direction, and my left ski in another.

After a minute or so, I tried to move, attempting to evaluate the damage.

Fortunately, the other person (whose mass was twice that of mine) wasn't injured.

The entire group was standing around me, bringing me my helmet and ski.

I tried to move. It appeared that my situation wasn't that bad. My neck and left hand hurt but I could still stand.

I thanked the group for their help and for bringing me my helmet and ski, and after they had gone, I tried to continue skiing.

I was being very careful, but I could still ski.

To avoid any future fear of skiing I continued for another hour or so.

That evening, and each of the following evenings I took a

therapeutic massage and participated in some physiotherapy. Each day, my neck and hand got better.

I learned another important lesson; you are not alone, your health and safety also depend on others. Those who are behind you and even those who are in front of you.

In addition to the downhill skiing, I did some cross-country skiing as well. My longest run was 10 kilometers, done at night, a somewhat unique experience. Only the two of us, in the light of a half-moon, with only the trees and the wind.

I was hoping that some cross-country skiing would help me to keep in shape for running, but it appears that different muscles are employed, so it probably hasn't contributed much (except for the pain in the muscles, that were not being used much before…).

But all in all, I can say that I enjoyed it greatly.

This time my rehabilitation went really quickly, mostly because of the excellent therapeutic massages and physiotherapy exercises I received from Magda, who used to be a professional skier and who was well acquainted with these types of injuries. Thanks Magda!

By my last day at Szklarska I was almost fully recovered, and ready for my next adventure.

March 19th, I'm back from my ski vacation.

Around 7A.M. I go on a 5km run. It takes me close to 32 minutes, much worse than my time two weeks earlier.

The next day, Wednesday I go for a swim, but only two kilometers and my time is very poor.

On Thursday, another slow run, and on Friday, a 20km bike ride, again my time is slow!

What has happened?!

Only a two-week ski break and my performance has dramatically deteriorated.

Maybe one of the reasons for the regression is that for those two weeks I used other muscles?

Or maybe, I should blame some lingering effects of the accident?!

In any case, I'm back to square one.

Well, maybe one and a half.

Conclusions:
- Vacation is great, but doesn't contribute to overall performance.
- After the vacation I have to work harder to get back to where I was before.

CHAPTER 3

•••••••••••••••

Meeting Sharks, Swimming and Diving Camp in Maldives

This year I planned to go skiing twice: the first time as I do usually, at the beginning of March, to Poland, and the second time a month later, in mid-April at Val Thorens in France.

Hopefully making some significant progress.

When Olivia, of Ori Sela's Water World, told me about a swimming and diving camp in Maldives that was to take place at the beginning of April, I replied: "no way, this year March and April are devoted to skiing."

But she signed me up anyway…

Swimming is my weakest point in the triathlon competitions, so "investing" in some improvement in this area sounded like a good idea.

And it was also an opportunity to get some personal direction from the inventor of the WEST swimming technique, the Maestro Ori Sela!

And as an additional "bonus," scuba diving in Maldives! Maybe even seeing some sharks or manta rays?!

It sounded like a dream!

There was room for only twenty swimmers on the Princess Dhonkamana liveaboard yacht.

I like to make quick decisions. My intuition said YES! And the very next day I confirm with Olivia that I am coming!

Despite it is taking place right in-between my two ski vacations...

I hope that my immune system can adjust quickly enough to these temperature changes from below zero in the mountains to the warm Indian Ocean and then back again to below zero weather...

The decision came just in time, as shortly thereafter all 20 rooms on the yacht were booked.

We arrive at the yacht on Sunday, March 31st, and without any delay, jump into the water.

During my 7 day stay on the Dhonkamana, we swam twice a day; a two-hour session in the morning and a shorter one, 45 minutes devoted mostly to the WEST swimming technique, in the afternoon.

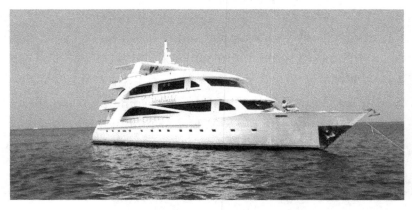

This was our "home" for that week.

In between swimming sessions we did some diving; 40 to 50 minutes under the water.

Already during the first swimming session Ori "diagnosed" my main problem of which I was already aware; during the catch stage my hands shouldn't cross the midline, I was doing that, especially with my right hand, without noticing.

Also, the angle of my palm wasn't straight back as it was supposed to be, which meant that in the catch stage of my stroke I was pushing less water and thus gaining less propulsion.

The third correction was to avoid moving the head as much as possible.

I began implementing these corrections and the effect was immediate, I swam easier and faster.

Although my primary goal in coming on the trip was to improve my swimming technique, I must admit that all in all it was a wonderful week.

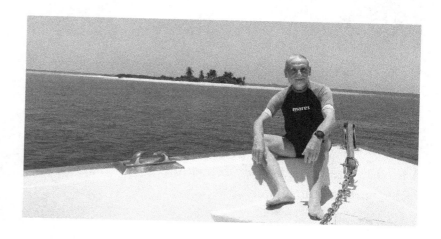

I very much enjoyed the diving, being in the middle of no-where, and the other people on the yacht. Being together 24/7, on the yacht and in the ocean, we quickly formed fast, friendly bonds. Swimming together, eating together, drinking (including some alcohol…) together and late night social gatherings lasting well past midnight.

Everybody was very sport-aware. Basically, all were swimmers (the vast majority much better than me), but several were also runners, including marathon runners, triathlon and one person – Igal, had completed an Iron Man Triathlon, several times!

On one of the dives I "met" this beautiful manta ray face-to-face!

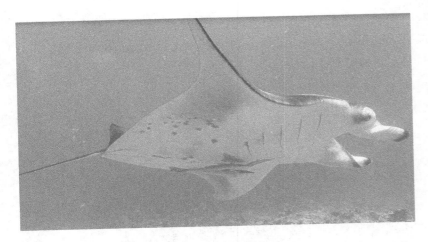

I was so overwhelmed I couldn't breathe.

I felt like she wanted to say something to me, maybe: like - "what are you doing here?!"

Before the next diving session, the divemaster told us that when she makes a particular sign, we shall all take hold of a stone or something solid and not move.

After 15 minutes or so of diving, the moment came. The divemaster made the sign and we all looked and couldn't believe what we were seeing; an endless pack of sharks was passing nearby, maybe 20 meters from us. We were by their side and it seemed that they had not yet noticed us.

In any case, they didn't seem to care and there were scores of sharks passing. Some were swimming in the opposite direction and it looked like street traffic.

These were long definitely unforgettable moments.

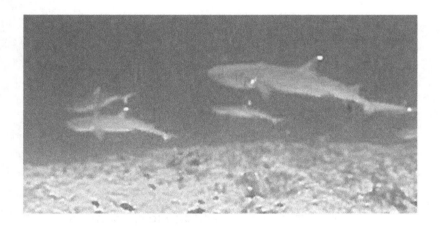

By April 8ᵀᴴ, following this amazing week, I was back home again.

I suddenly felt a strong urge to run!

Despite having landed at 5 PM, I didn't feel like going to sleep.

After organizing my things a bit and a quick shower, I ran an initial "opening" 5 kilometers. It was not one of my fastest runs, but it was easy.

I had twelve days left until my ski trip to Val Thorens in the French Alps, so I didn't want to miss a day of exercise; running, swimming, biking.

On April 19th, the day before my flight, the summary of my sport activities was as follows:

Running three times a week:

5 kilometers – intervals running, reaching 4:30/km!

6 kilometers – tempo run (designed to improve endurance), usually around 5:45/km

7km LSD (Long Slow Distance), 6:20/km

It sums up more or less to 18kms/week. At this pace it will reach 80kms/month.

All in all, the runs go quite easily, with great joy and pleasure. The knee is okay most of the time, but when it hurts, even a bit, I start to panic…

But usually that passes very quickly.

I very much hope that the next ski vacation will not put me back.

To motivate myself even more, and also to check my progress, I sign up for a 10km run which is to take place in Herziliya on Saturday, May 4th, less than a week after I return from the ski trip.

This will be my first 10K run, since September and the last injury.

CHAPTER 4

....

Back to White, Another Ski Week, Val Thorens, France

Despite its being almost the end of the ski season, the last week of April, the conditions are quite good. Only the strong winds are a less pleasant.

This village in the French region of Rhone-Alpes which lies at an altitude of 2,300 meters, offers views of the French as well as the Swiss and Italian Alps, and is regarded as the highest skiing station in Europe.

Les Trois Vallees, the 3 Valleys ski area is known as the largest connected skiing region in the world, with its three valleys and approximately 600 kilometers of slopes. At Val Thorens alone there is a selection of almost 70 slopes covering 140 kilometers, well connected by 30 ski lifts.

For me it was more challenging than skiing in Poland as the slopes were steeper and longer. But I managed quite well and noted further improvement.

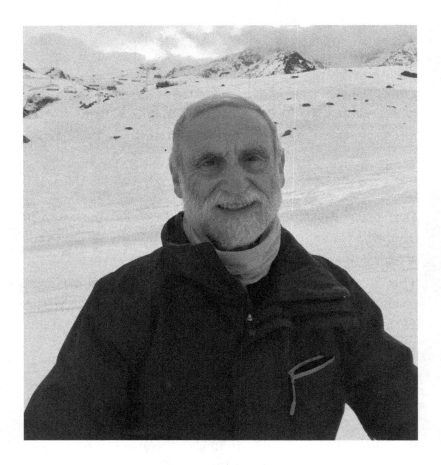

I was very careful, not to end-up with another injury, so I took fewer risks and skied mostly on the green and blue slopes (the beginner and intermediate slopes), still enjoying myself very much.

I came home on Sunday, April 28th at 4am, slept three hours and then went for a "refreshing" run.

3.7kms, pace 5:47, easy.

CHAPTER 5
················
A Surprising Race, Running My First 10km Since the Injury.

I have less than a week left to prepare for the 10K, so I run the 5.7kms intervals run the next day – the average pace is 5:13, my best ever! Average HBR is 161, maximum HBR is 179.

I take a one-day break from running and go to swim in the pool – 2.4kms with a slight improvement in speed.

On Wednesday I run 8.6 kilometers at 5:31/km, which is slower than the intervals run. I am not able to push myself harder and am disappointed. It's good enough for a reasonable finish time but not enough for a medal.

The following two days I rest in order to accumulate more energy and glycogen in my muscles and liver.

But on Friday afternoon out of the blue, I feel a sudden, unexpected pain in my lower back. I have no idea what triggered it.

I try self-massaging with Arnica cream – That doesn't help.

Some stretching, lying down, standing, lying down again.

The pain is still there.

I take a hot bath, I soak in hot water for 20 minutes, the pain decreases slightly.

I get a small sample of Perskindol, a local pain relief gel. I apply a small amount and go to meditate.

After the meditation, three hours since the pain started, it has almost passed.

Another hour and it has disappeared entirely.

Seems that I will be able run tomorrow!

But what was it?! Some kind of warning?!

On Saturday I wake up early, at 4:30 am. By 6:00 I am in Herziliya. The weather is good, after two very hot days, the temperature has dropped to 17 degrees Celsius. For average temperatures in Israel for May, this is low.

I feel some pent up energy and have a good start. After two kilometers my Garmin fitness tracker reads 10:05, at a pace of 5:03 a kilometer– fantastic!

But I begin to feel the strain and have to slow down a bit.

After 5 kilometers my average pace is 5:15/km.

I notice that I'm slowing down below this, so I push myself to shorten the "interval" and succeed in maintaining this pace.

I finish at 52:33, my best 10K ever, my pace per kilometer - 5:15. Maximum heart rate is 183, which is reasonable, and after three minutes it drops quickly to level out at ≈100.

Herziliya is a fast, professional run, and my 52:33 gives me only 9th place out of 23 in my age category and around 850th place out of 1,700 – which is exactly in the middle of the overall ranking.

It was the first 10k that I had run in 8 months, since the last one that I ran in September, while recovering from the partial tear of the patellar tendon. Much earlier than I had originally planned.

I was tired, but satisfied.

CHAPTER 6
· · · · · · · · · · · · · · · ·
On the Wave!

Back to Tamarindo and surfing, May 11th – May 23rd

I was in Tamarindo, Costa Rica, two years ago, and it was my best surfing vacation ever. I'm quite an amateur surfer and seek easy waves. That means, not too high, 3 to 4 feet, but long and predictable. I mean, that I'm able to see the coming wave, to paddle to it, and even if my pop-up isn't perfect, to have another fraction of a second to correct my stance.

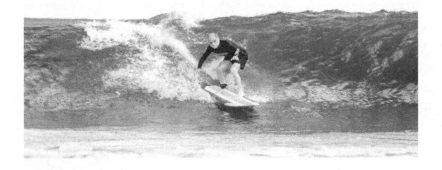

Tamarindo hasn't disappointed, and I surfed some very nice

waves, even a bit bigger than I had planned.

I love the feeling when I sense the wave, pop-up and "fly" with it. It is short, 10 seconds. 15 to 20 seconds at most. Maybe because it is such a short moment of time, it means so much to me.

I also went diving. It was my best diving experience, sharks, mantas and a lot of fish.

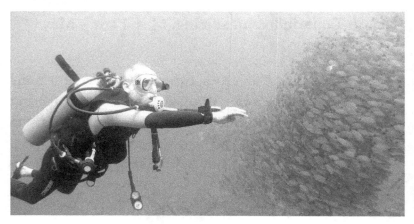

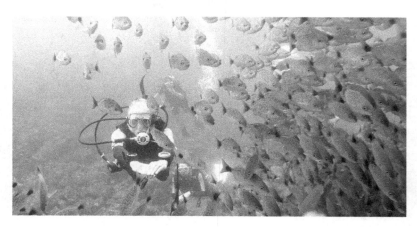

And beautiful views!

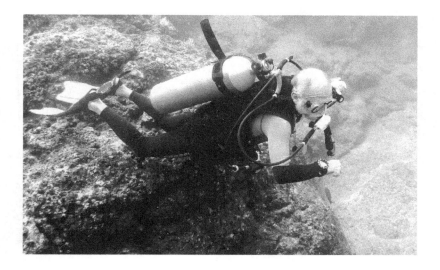

I was only 17 meters below the surface, but the view looking down was like that of the Grand Canyon!

I also felt an improvement in my diving technique; I remained very calm and used less oxygen. I felt that I was maintaining good self-control.

When the morning tide was very low and there were no waves, I went for a run.

In Tamarindo, on May 21st I ran 10,150 meters with a lot of up-hills and downhills. Pace 6:11/km, good enough. Max HR 171.

CHAPTER 7

····················

Back on Track!

In May and June, I began increasing my distances:

On May 26th 10,340 meters, pace 6.14/km, max HR 168

On May 29th 10,600 meters pace 6:58/km, max HR 162 only!

The 6:58min/km was my slowest pace, but it was a hot day, 23 degrees Celsius, and only 48 hours since the other 10K+ run.

Based on how I felt, I set up the following plan:

Running three times a week

- Intervals on Saturdays, staying in the 5-6km range
- Tempo on Mondays, staying in the 7-8km range
- LSD on Wednesdays, increasing 300 – 500 meters each week. Since the intervals will be on Saturdays, this will give my body 72 hours to recover from the long run. (LSD stands for long slow distance…)

This would come to 23-24kms/week in the near future and 25-26kms/week by July or August, leading to ≈100km/month. I'll try not to exceed the 100km/month, remembering the partial tear in the patellar tendon that happened when I was running 125km/month last summer.

100km/month is not much for one who wants to compete in a half-marathon, but I believe my approach of emphasizing **quality running** over the "brute force" approach - emphasizing the quantity – the number of kilometers, as the key parameter, should work well for me.

In my running philosophy, the right balance between effort and rest, the right nutrition in general and "fueling" during the run, (taking an energy gel packet or eating a date) while swimming and biking on the other days, should enable me to run farther and faster.

Running in July and August

During the months of July and August, the very hot Israeli summer, I run early in the morning. I begin my runs before 6 AM, but even that early the temperature is at least 27 degrees Celsius.

Following the partial tear of my patellar tendon last July, when I was running 125 km per month, I didn't want to run more than 100kms/month. So, while increasing the long run by 500 meters each week, I kept the other two runs fixed: intervals – 5kms and tempo - 7kms.

During June I succeeded in keeping it to 100 kilometers, but by July and August it eventually reached 110kms/month.

But I was running slower and never on subsequent days. The weekly program was bike-run-swim-run-swim-bike-run, and seems that it worked out quite well.

On June 5th I began with the over 10K runs, running my first 11km run since my injury a year earlier.

The 12km run occurred a bit ahead of schedule, but conditions in Cambridge where I was staying at the time, were so ideal, that I couldn't resist the temptation (the temperature was only 15 degrees Celsius).

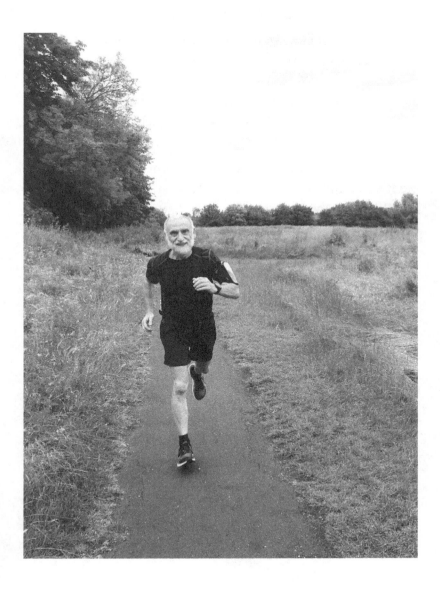

It went quite smoothly and I very much enjoyed running surrounded by the beautiful Cambridge scenery.

I had come to Cambridge to attend the wedding of my son Avishai with Estherina. Avishai was at Cambridge completing post-doctorate research in astrophysics.

As a bonus I got the opportunity to run in the most perfect scenario and conditions.

After coming back to Israel, my plans crystalized: adding 500 meters every week until September 4th when I would reach 18kms.

I suffered from two orthopaedic problems: the twice-injured right knee and the left forefoot. At least I was balanced, one problem for each leg. ☺

With the knee problem I coped by softening the foot "landing" as much as possible, by reducing the overall amount of weekly running – keeping it at no more than 25 – 27kms and wearing more cushioned running shoes. The Altra Paradigm 3, and later Paradigm 4.5 were much heavier (319 grams/shoe), than the so pleasant and fast Escalante (200 grams/shoe), and it slowed my pace by some 10 percent.

With the forefoot problem I coped by constantly focusing on correct leg movement, landing softly, staying on the ground as briefly as possible and pulling the leg back as soon as it touched the road. Also, the cushioned Paradigm running shoes helped.

Still, it happened that after running 12 to 13 kilometers my level of pain on a scale of 0 to 10 would reach between 4 and 5. But I was used to running with pain, and the problem with my forefoot wasn't a "deal breaker."

Regarding the knee it was different. Every time the pain showed up, even as low as 2 to 3 I was in a kind of panic.

The orthopaedists told me not to run and warned me, that the damage might be irreversible.

And I had already lost half of the meniscus...

But my love of running was greater than my mathematical, logical, rational thinking...

I added to my weekly training more strengthening exercises, like squats, believing that the stronger all of my muscles were, the lesser would be the pressure on the tendons.

In general, this worked out reasonably for me, at least most of the time.

CHAPTER 8
· · · · · · · · · · · · · · · ·
The Riddle of My Left Forefoot Pain

The pain in my left forefoot has been with me as long as I can remember, and usually it appears after a long walk. It is also linked to which shoes I am wearing.

The forefoot is the anterior area of the foot. It is composed of the five metatarsal bones, the fourteen phalanges and associated soft tissue structures. It is a common site of pathology in podiatry.

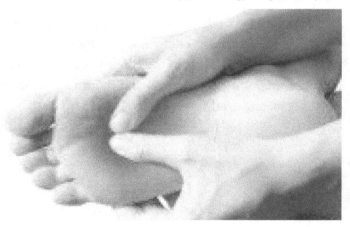

One of the more extreme cases I can recall was in Warsaw. I was taking a walk on a winter evening, it was minus ten degrees (Celsius) and the pain was so bad that I had to stop, take my shoe off and massage my left forefoot - I couldn't stand the pain!

I have tried various shoes and have found that Rockport shoes are the most comfortable for me. They seem to delay the onset of pain.

I have also tried various insoles, some of which eased the pain a little bit.

But when I started running longer distances, the pain became quite severe. Not at the beginning of the run, but after 5 to 6 kilometers.

I visited an orthopedist. He wasn't able to help me but he recommended that I try a podiatrist.

A podiatrist, also known as a podiatric physician, is a medical professional devoted to the treatment of disorders of the foot, ankle, and lower extremity.

I approached two. Their consensus was that the source of the problem was a bunion, a deformity of the joint connecting the big toe to the foot. The big toe often bends towards the other toes and the joint becomes red and painful. The onset of bunions is typically gradual.

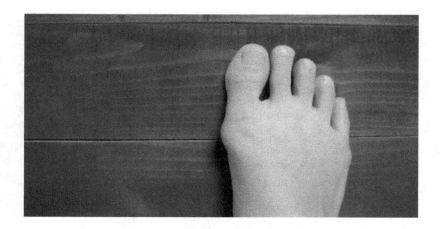

I guessed that the problem was related to the once very fashionable narrow shape of elegant dress shoes. At one time I was wearing such shoes and I now believe that they could have been the source of my bunion.

The diagnosis was that the bunion had caused bursitis in my foot.

Bursitis is the inflammation of one or more bursae (small sacs) of synovial fluid in the body. They are lined with a synovial membrane that secretes a lubricating synovial fluid. There are more than 150 bursae in the human body. The bursae rest at the points where internal functionaries, such as muscles and tendons, slide across bone. Healthy bursae create a smooth, almost frictionless functional gliding surface making normal movement painless. When bursitis occurs, however, movement relying on the inflamed bursa becomes difficult and painful. Moreover, movement of tendons and muscles over the inflamed bursa aggravates its inflammation, perpetuating the problem. Muscle can also be stiffened.

One of the podiatrists I visited suggested surgery. I refused. I wasn't convinced that this would solve the problem and the outcome is quite unpredictable.

But I was lucky. While shopping for new running shoes I entered "Marathon," a small shop, offering reasonable prices, that specializes in running shoes.

It wasn't "love at first sight." Eliezer, the owner, who was once a marathon runner and coach, seemed quite "indifferent" to my plight. But I liked the fact that he offered to let me to try out shoes on a treadmill, while making a video to analyze my running.

He also suggested that I try on a pair of Altra running shoes.

For me, this was love at first sight, or first stride.

They felt so good on me that I didn't want to take them off. Altra Running Shoes have several advantages over other running shoes, but the key one for me, which changed my life, and in particular my running, was the very wide toe-box, which offered the room that I needed for my forefoot.

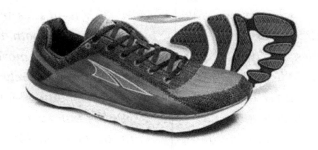

Initially I used them only for running, but I soon noticed that switching to other shoes was bringing back the pain in my forefoot, the inflammation.

Eventually I gave up all other shoes, bought 5 pairs of various models of Altra and am now wearing only these for all occasions (except the Cambridge wedding of my son Avishai & Estherina).

The situation has dramatically improved. I can now run longer distances with no pain. Only after about 8 kilometers does the pain start to return.

But if I can run those 8 kilometers with no pain, it means that the problem isn't permanent!

My mathematical-logical thinking led me to a clear conclusion: if the pain increases with time, the problem must be in the repetitive movement!

Probably there is a small imperfection in my stride. I don't feel it while running short distances, but after repeating the move 8,000 times, it begins to hurt (I do 160 – 170 strides per minute, 8 kilometers takes me some 48 minutes, so 48 minutes X 165=≈8,000.

Incidentally, in one of his excellent Chi Running lessons, Danny Dreyer was talking about the problem of "toeing-off." I immediately realized what was happening: I was toeing off my toes!

There is a common misunderstanding about the function of toes in running. Their only purpose in running is maintaining balance/stabilization and the feeling of support. Pushing off actively with our toes leads to various disorders and pain in the foot.

So, we should mainly bend the knees and lift the ankles – not push ourselves off!

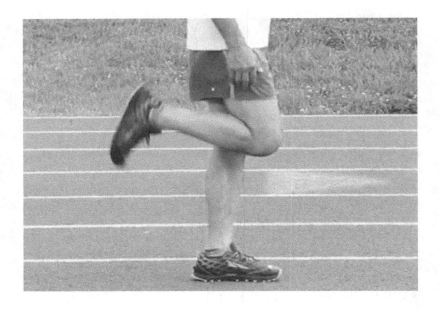

On June 26th 2019, on my 13km run, my key focus was to visualize lifting the ankles instead of toeing-off.

It was the run with the least amount of pain ever in the forefoot, in an over 10K run! The first 10km were painless, and then the pain was at level 1, after 11 kilometers at level 2, and by the end it had reached to level 3 (on a scale of from 0 to 10).

I felt, that I was about to solve the most disturbing problem in my long runs and the key obstacle for my running a half marathon or longer!

Needless to say, I was very happy!

CHAPTER 9
·················
Running at Night

At the beginning of July, I deviated for one week from my Master Plan, and participated in the 10K Nitzan Night Run. "Nitzan" is an organization, with the charter of raising awareness of a much neglected subject - learning disabilities and ADHD (Attention Deficit Hyperactivity Disorder).

The slogan of the run was: "Running for success," following the belief, that everyone has the right to realize his/her potential.

It wasn't one of my fastest runs, but I enjoyed it very much. I like night runs.

CHAPTER 10

My First 16K Run

On August 7th for the first time in my life, I ran 16 kilometers.

From that time on, each week would be a new distance record.

It took me one hour and fifty minutes, but at the end I really didn't feel exhausted. Actually, I felt that I could keep on running!

It was one of my best runs and I felt light and happy.

I do not recognize myself since the metamorphosis three years ago. But I like my new self.

I loved the experience, the way I felt at the end and my sense of satisfaction.

CHAPTER 11
•••••••••••••••••
Running 17K for the First Time!

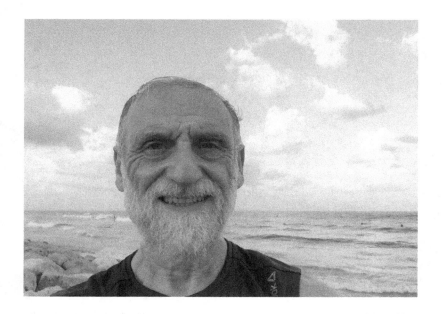

Running had become a key ingredient in my life and happiness!

In the long runs I treated myself with two "meals": a gel (100 calories and some electrolytes) after 5 kilometers and a date (50 calories) after 10 kilometers.

Not that I was hungry, just in case, to make sure there is enough sugar in my blood.

Later, when I reached 15 kilometers, I added another date, so it was date-gel-date.

After 10 kilometers I also took an electrolyte tablet, to replenish all the salts I was losing by sweating.

I was running with a small hydration backpack.

I was drinking about 1 liter of water for every 10 kilometers, 1.5 liters for every 15 kilometers, etc.

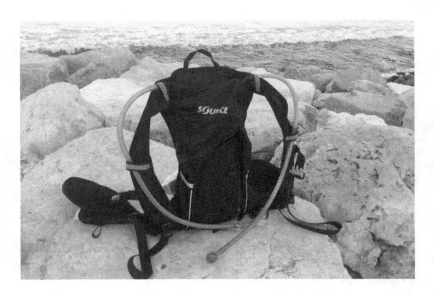

On August 21st I ran 17 kilometers for the first time. I love this number!

It was like being on a journey... There were moments when there were no thoughts, like when meditating, sometimes there were thoughts related to the run, and sometimes there were other thoughts...

The last two kilometers were more difficult than usual, but I like challenges.

The average pace was 7 minutes and 12 seconds per kilometer, quite slow. That's because I was being a bit cautious in the first half of the run, keeping an energy reserve of for the second half, and the high heat and humidity made it even more difficult.

CHAPTER 12

·················

A Surprise in the Sea!

One day I was swimming in the sea. My usual training distance, 1,500 to 1,600 meters.

I swim out some 750 to 800 meter in one direction and then back to the beach.

It isn't always accurate, as I am unable to swim in a perfectly straight line and frequently my sea path becomes a triangle, which can add as much as 100 to 200 meters to the originally planned distance.

The sea was a bit choppy, actually it was at the maximum wave height that I allow myself to swim in, 70 centimeters.

But it was still okay for me.

When I swim in the sea, I do not raise my head very often, as raising your head slows you down. I was looking down at the bottom, it wasn't very deep, so I could see the seabed and some small fish.

I had reached a distance of some 800 meters (as measured by my GPS watch) and began to turn around.

After a few minutes I raised my head.

It was a weird view.

It took me a second or two to understand what I was seeing.

Rocks!

A few meters ahead of me.

I wasn't supposed to be there.

Suddenly I understood. It was the strong current pushing me towards the rocks! Like prey, thrown into the cage of a hungry animal.

But why would Neptune want to sacrifice me to the rocks?!

What had I done wrong to offend him?!

I began paddling strongly in the opposite direction.

But I didn't move.

I stayed in the same place.

The current was stronger than me.

Of course, no man can fight the powers of nature.

I tried to paddle even harder, the hardest I could.

It didn't help, I began slowly approaching the rocks and any strong wave would throw me onto them!

Luckily despite the feeling of panic my brain hadn't froze up and I could still think.

I'm a mathematician, logic… intuition

Yes, probably this was intuition, or my subconsciousness, that was telling me what to do. It was saying: "Don't try to swim against the current, you have no chance, this strategy is hopeless. But you can swim vertically, 90 degrees to the current!"

Yes, this strategy began to work.

Still paddling the strongest and the fastest that I could, I began to slowly and gradually escape from the rocks…

I had survived once again, thanks Neptune for sparing my life!

From all that I could have learned from this happy-ending "drama," my conclusion was to raise my head more often.

CHAPTER 13
....
Passing the Test

In August I took an extensive series of fitness tests. The results were outstanding, I was in perfect physical shape.

But, after the tests, the ECG electrodes were still on me, and surprisingly they showed that my heart "missed two beats."

Appears that this phenomenon of Premature Atrial Contractions (PACs) is quite common among long distance runners.

Since it happened during the recovery period, following a perfect ECG reading during a half hour effort, I wasn't very much worried.

But it still had a psychological effect, and the next day, during a normal run, I started to feel some pain in my chest…

It was recommended to me that I go see a cardiologist, take an echocardiogram test and even use a Holter monitor (a portable device that continuously measures and records your heart's activity) for at least 24 hours.

I also got a certificate, that I could compete in triathlons and long runs, and I was happy.

Regarding the heart tests, I decided to postpone them and see whether or not my heart continued to complain.

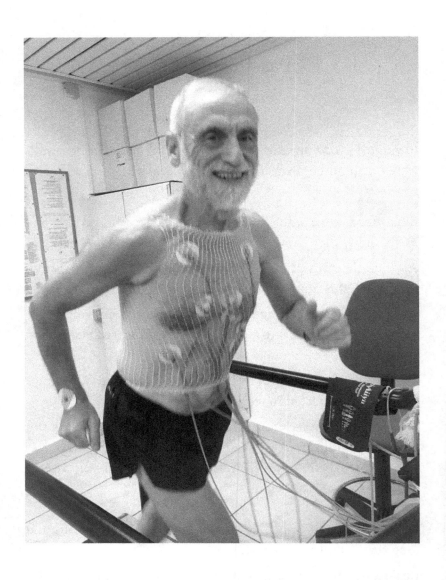

CHAPTER 14

····················

My Sport-Influenced Nutrition

Proper nutrition is a key part of succeeding in sport activities and in competitions.

The others are: training, technique, determination and a strong mind.

What do we need to eat to enable our body to perform at its best?

Definitely calories and carbohydrates are not an issue.

Neither are fats.

We need a decent amount of proteins. The consensus is around 0.8gr multiplied by the body weight.

In my case 60X0.8=48grams.

But this amount should be increased in proportion to the intensity and timing of your workouts. There is no exact formulas, but by adding roughly from 20 up to 50 percent.

In my case 70 grams per day should be more than enough.

The other "challenge" is vitamins and minerals.

Vitamins are readily available in fruits, salads and nuts (the B group or vitamin B complex), so they shouldn't be a problem.

To get the right numerous minerals depends very much on **the**

diversification of our diet.

Obviously, if we eat a lot of "empty" calories (e.g. carbohydrates like bread, ice-cream, cookies etc.), we may be lacking some of the minerals, or do not get an adequate amount of them.

What is the role of these minerals?

First the electrolytes.

Electrolytes are minerals necessary for conducting electricity (transmitting nerve impulses) in the body.

Other key functions of electrolytes include maintaining water balance and helping muscles (including the heart) contract and relax.

The key electrolytes are **sodium, potassium and chloride.**

During intensive sport activity we sweat and lose electrolytes along with water.

I must tell you a story. When I began running longer distances, especially on the hot days of the Israeli summer (when temperatures average 30 degrees Celsius or 86 degrees Fahrenheit) and sweated a lot, I noticed that after the run I had a craving for olives!

No, I wasn't pregnant (I'm a man).

After this happened a few more times, I came to a conclusion: I sweated a lot and therefore lost salt – the body demands salt (sodium & chloride)!

Since then, after sweating I do take a few olives.

The potassium I get from bananas.

More specifically about the function of these electrolytes.

Potassium is responsible for regulating heartbeat and muscle function and it is important in neuron function. The daily recommended intake is relatively high – at least 3.5 grams, and it is not easy to "collect" this amount.

Extremely high or low potassium levels can cause an irregular heartbeat, which can be fatal.

Sodium regulates the total amount of water in the body and maintains the proper functioning of the nervous, muscular, and other systems.

Chloride helps maintain a normal balance of body fluids.

The required amounts of these minerals are not large; 1 to 3 grams per day.

Sodium and chloride are easily available as salt, but getting the required amount of potassium (3.5grams/day) is more difficult.

Good sources of potassium are potatoes baked with the skin, beans and lentils, broccoli, pistachio and the best known and preferred by athletes – the banana.

The other key minerals are calcium, phosphorus, magnesium, iron and zinc.

Calcium

Calcium is the most abundant mineral in our body and performs a number of basic functions.

99% of the body's calcium serves to keep our bones and teeth strong.

The rest of the calcium in our body plays key roles in cell signaling, blood clotting, muscle contraction and nerve functioning.

Cells use calcium to activate certain enzymes, transport ions across the cellular membrane, and send and receive neurotransmitters during communication with other cells.

As an electrolyte, calcium is also one of the key players in maintaining a regular heartbeat, but too much calcium is not good for the heart, so we should be careful if taking a calcium supplement.

Phosphorus

Phosphorus is an essential mineral necessary for energy production, being a key component of ATP (Adenosine triphosphate) - "the energy currency of the body" in all living organisms.

ATPs are readily used to fuel many functions in the body, one example being muscle contraction.

Other key functions of phosphorus are in growth and repair of body cells and tissues.

Magnesium

Magnesium, an abundant mineral in the body, is naturally present in many foods.

Magnesium is a cofactor in more than 300 enzyme systems that regulate diverse biochemical reactions in the body, including protein synthesis, muscle and nerve function, blood glucose control, and blood pressure regulation.

Magnesium is necessary for energy production.

It contributes to the structural development of bone and is required for the synthesis of DNA.

Magnesium also plays a role in the active transport of calcium and potassium ions across cell membranes, a process that is important to nerve impulse conduction, muscle contraction, and normal heart rhythm.

Iron

One of the most important functions of iron is in heme synthesis, which forms hemoglobin, a protein found in red blood cells.

Hemoglobin's primary role is to transport oxygen from the lungs to body tissues to maintain basic life functions. Without healthy red blood cells, our body can't get enough oxygen and this can result in feeling increasingly tired or exhausted.

Iron is necessary for immune cells proliferation and maturation, particularly lymphocytes, which are associated with helping us to keep healthy. Lower iron levels may contribute to an increased risk of our immune systems being compromised and our bodies falling sick.

Zinc

Zinc plays an important part in many biological processes. It plays a key role during physiological growth and fulfills an immune function. It is vital for the functionality of more than 300 enzymes, for the stabilization of DNA, and for gene expression.

Crucial for health and metabolism.

To summarize; we need only a few grams of each mineral, since the body uses these micro-nutrients on a molecular level and each gram of a mineral contains trillions of trillions of molecules, which flow in the blood and can reach everywhere.

To solve the mathematical-nutrition equation of getting enough proteins and some key minerals, I invented **THE BAL MEAL!**

The full recipe of the secret BAL meal is disclosed here for the first time.

The BAL MEAL (Beans and Lentils) is my main daily meal.

It took me over a year and a lot of experimenting, to reach the perfect balance between nutritional values and taste.

The main goal was to build a meal, which would provide the major chunk of proteins and minerals, based on the assumption that I get enough vitamins from salads and fruits.

I tried a broad variety of beans and lentils and the four left in the final recipe were chosen based mainly on taste, as the nutritional value of most beans and lentils is quite similar.

You are invited to do your own experimentation and pick your own winning combination.

The preparation process comprises of two steps:

- Cooking the key ingredients (B&L) and the beetroot
- The lunch time preparation

I usually cook enough of the beans and lentils to last for 4 to 5 days, as the cooking of some of them requires time: the lentils 10 to 15 minutes after the water comes to a boil (use plenty of water), the mung beans take 20 minutes and the kidney beans around 40 minutes, but following 12 hours of soaking in boiled but cool water.

I begin by heating a frying pan with a small amount of olive oil, just enough to cover the bottom.

After a few minutes I begin adding the ingredients, one by one, chopped into tiny pieces, to avoid too strong of a taste of any one ingredient.

Starting with the roots, since they require more time to cook before they are edible.

I begin with nice fresh Celeriac, or celery root.

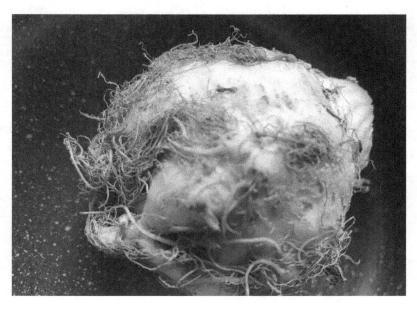

Half of this forms one serving.

I then add parsley root, a small cube of ginger, half an onion, and some garlic and curcumin.

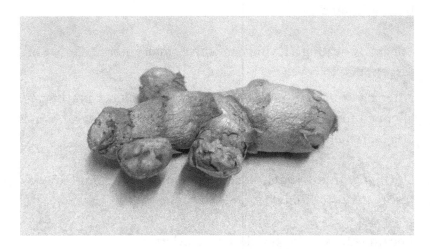

The curcumin (see above) is cut into tiny pieces.

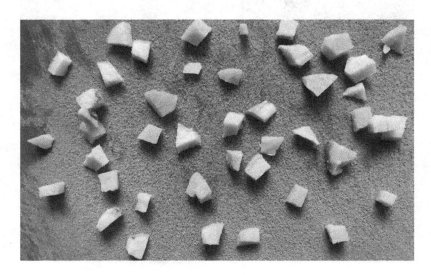

If no fresh curcumin is available then I use Turmeric powder.

All the roots are chopped into tiny pieces to allow for good "blending" - mixing and to avoid too strong a taste.

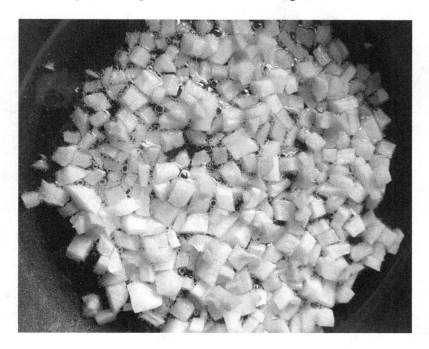

The first layer is ready!

Now add some tofu (I usually use 50 to 70 grams), and beetroot (one third to a half, depending on how big it is).

Also the beetroot is cooked in advance for 2 to 3 days.

I cook it for about 40 minutes.

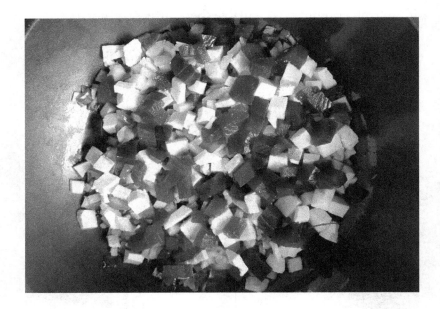

I add a lot of spices: Himalayan salt, black pepper, red paprika, parsley, dill, cumin, basil, oregano and of course garlic. Adding 3 to 4 spices to each layer.

You can use turmeric powder, if no fresh curcumin is available.

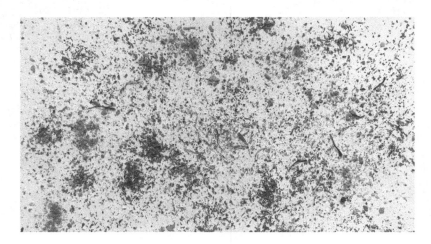

The "10 seasonings" composition.

Add 10 to 15 threads of saffron.

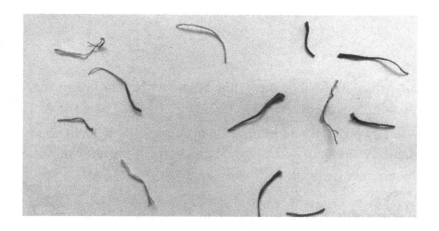

Last to be added are the beans and lentils: red lentils, green lentils, mung beans and kidney beans.

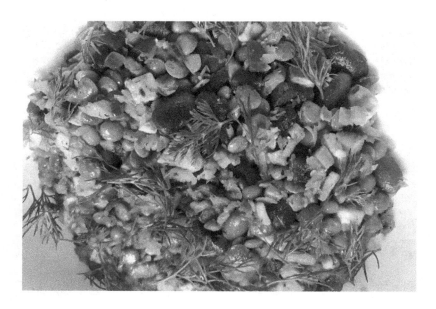

Add dill and parsley to the four beans and lentils .

Lunch is served!

~

So, what do we end up with, after all the hard work and preparations?

A lot of protein – 34 grams, for me almost 70 percent of my daily requirement and a significant chunk of my daily mineral requirement as well.

Below is a detailed summary of the protein and the key minerals in the BAL meal:

	Weight	Proteins	Potassium	Calcium	Phosphorus	Magnesium	Iron	Zinc
			Values for cooked, actual amounts in one serving (400 gr)					
Red lentils	80	7.2	243	17	107	21	2.7	1.3
Tofu	75	12.8	132	203	132	35	1.1	0.8
Green lentils	50	4.5	154	9	64	11	1.5	0.8
Mung beans	45	4.8	113	12	33	17	0.6	0.2
Beetroot	40	0.7	130	6	16	9	0.3	0.2
Onion	40	0.4	58	9	12	4	0.1	0.1
Celery root	20	0.4	60	9	23	4	0.1	0.1
Kidney beans	25	2.3	141	14	41	14	0.8	0.3
Ginger	10	0.2	42	2	3	4	0.1	0.0
Parsley root	10	0.2	56	5	7	4	0.1	0.1
Curcumin	5	0.4	126	9	13	10	2.1	0.2
Total, mg		34g	1,255	295	451	133	10	4
RDA		50	3,500	1,000	700	420	18	11
% of RDA		68%	36%	29%	64%	32%	53%	37%

RDA = Recommended Dietary Allowance

The key is diversity – a little bit of everything.

The other major meal is either rice, or pasta (but not both.)

And of course, the daily salad: tomato, cucumber, sweet (red) pepper (full of vitamin C), a shallot onion, radish, the juice of one lemon and olive oil.

On occasion I may add some nuts, but not really a lot. Not always and usually only to one of the day's meals.

Between the meals I eat fruits – one full fruit in season or two halves of two different fruits (in season).

I do have my "sins"; I usually end the day with soy cream, 120 calories, but almost 4 grams of protein and 150 milligrams of calcium.

During the day, another "sin" of mine is green or white tea with two small "industrial" oatmeal cookies, ≈100 calories, no nutritional value.

CHAPTER 15

Food Supplements.

I'm well aware, that there are no simple conclusions regarding the benefits of food supplements.

But the question is what is the question…?

If one expects a food supplement to cure cancer or to improve memory, then the research is a waste of time. No food supplement can create such a miracle.

But if you are aware of what may be missing from your diet on any one day, then a food supplement can be the perfect solution.

On a rest day, I usually don't take any supplements, except for B-12, which I take at least every other day, because as a vegan I have no natural means for acquiring it, and B-12 is crucial to many body and brain functions.

If I think, that on a specific day I may have not enough calcium, I'll take that supplement. The same for iron, potassium and zinc.

For me the key food supplements are some amino acids.

Let me explain.

There is a consensus that it is necessary to supply the body with between 50 and 70 grams of protein each day.

But measuring only the quantity of the protein is not quite accurate. There is also a major issue regarding the "quality" of the protein we get in food, especially its completeness.

During the digestive process the body decomposes protein into its basic building blocks, or the amino acids, which in turn float through the blood stream.

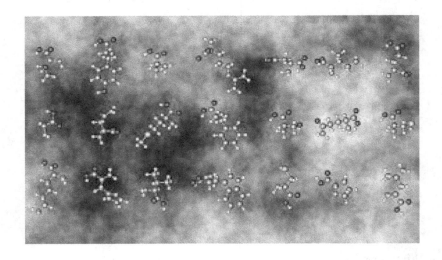

The chemical structure of the 20 amino acids.

Our physiological proteins consist of many instances (or sequences) of 20 different amino acids. The average protein is a chain of a few hundred of these 20 "letters."

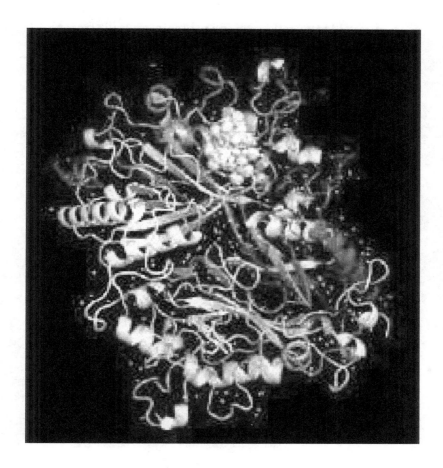

A beautiful protein

Each protein that is available in the food we eat is comprised of some of these amino acids, but usually not all twenty.

Therefore, we may have the required amount of proteins, but the composition, or decomposition, may be lacking in some amino acids.

From the bloodstream the amino acids are taken up into our

cells and inside the cells, specific proteins are built from these amino acids, according to the "instructions" in the cell's DNA.

The machine, which constructs the proteins from the amino-acids available in the cells, is the ribosome. There are many ribosomes within each living cell.

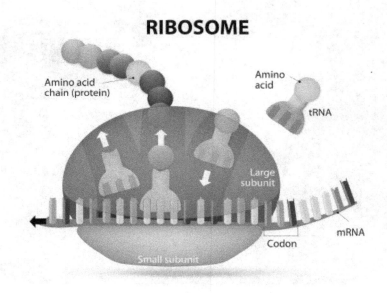

But if some amino-acids are missing, the ribosome can't fulfil its mission.

So actually, what we need to get from our food are the 20 amino acids.

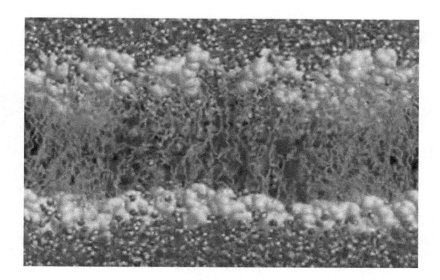

Another view of proteins and amino-acids.

It should be mentioned, that the amount of the various amino-acids is not equal.

On average it is 2 to 3 grams of each, but some are more abundant and some are rare and even half a gram could be enough.

To make sure I do have enough of each, even the rare ones, I take some amino-acid food supplements:

L-arginine, L-lysine L-carnitine and the three BCAA branched-chain Amino Acids (leucine, isoleucine and valine).

To summarize; it requires some effort to make sure that we are provided with all that we need, but on the other hand, our body is quite "tolerant" and even if it doesn't get everything, it can still perform quite well.

CHAPTER 16
••••••••••••••••••

Fueling the Body During and After the Workout

In a sport activity we burn from 5 to 10 calories per minute, depending on the length of the activity and its intensity.

Obviously, we have significant reserves, but for activities that last longer than an hour it is necessary to "re-fuel" the body.

My rule of thumb is to supply myself with some sugar every half hour.

I use dates (50 calories) and GU energy gel (100 calories) interchangeably. I.e. after the first half hour I take a gel, then after another half hour a date, etc.

Following the activity I usually eat a peanut butter cracker sandwich, or a Nature Valley protein bar (both contain about 10 grams of protein). And several olives.

Thus, my daily 2,000 calories diet increases on workout days to 2,200 up to 2,500, depending on the type of activity and in proportion to its length and intensity.

I aim at having the BAL meal inside a "two-hour-window,"

counting from the end of the activity.

Practically it is always after one and a half to two hours, given the after-workout starching, driving home and the meal preparations.

Summary

Initially some thought has to be devoted to this sport-oriented nutrition, but soon it will become a habit, and become "second nature" to you.

Actually, *these guidelines and an understanding of the body's needs is good and applicable for maintaining one's health whether or not you are involved in sport activities.*

CHAPTER 17
....
An Unexpected Twist in the Plot

Since my colorectal cancer 18 years ago, once a year I take a standard blood test with two markers that can indicate the possibility of a recurrence.

During the last 18 years the blood test has always gone smoothly with no issues.

Also, this time, it looked the same. But with a second look, the markers…

Yes, both markers had risen sharply; CA 19-9 from 14 to 38, an increase of 150 percent, leaving only a 5 percent probability that there was no relapse.

CEA had risen from 3.3 to 6, an increase of 80 percent, leaving less than a 5 percent chance that I was still free of cancer.

Combining both, it left less than a 1 percent probability that the cancer hadn't come back!

I consulted with several specialists. They all agreed that I should repeat the tests in a few weeks and in the meantime continue my life as usual and to enjoy myself.

At least I was being given a few weeks.

But it didn't make sense: I was physically very active, felt perfect, had healthy nutrition, what could have gone wrong?!

I began searching for an explanation and spoke with some of my wise friends. We looked for possibilities that the markers could increase in a healthy individual.

We soon found four research articles.

My friend Tehilla found the most important one: one that reported a significant increase in the markers following intensive sport activities!

This definitely looked like an explanation for my case!

Since I had planned to spend four days meditating, I decided to repeat the tests the day immediately following this retreat.

After all, my not being active for four consecutive days doesn't happen very frequently ...

The other studies described cases of inflammation, nutritional issues and drinking a lot of tea!

The tea case looked like a joke, but the person in the study with elevated markers had undergone every possible imaging test, and there was no sign of cancer.

Then, they noticed that she drank a lot of tea (1.5 liters/day) and asked her to stop for a few days. The markers' readings dropped dramatically.

Then, for the purpose of comparison, she was asked to go back to her regular habit and to drink a lot of tea. The markers rose again!

I do (actually I did at the time of the tests...) drink 4 to 5 cups of tea a day.

Not as much as the person in that study, but also my markers weren't as high as hers.

Suffice it to say that before repeating the blood tests, I abstained from tea.

From the day I got the initial results, actually from the moment that I understood that all signs seem to indicate that my cancer had returned, it was very tough.

Although usually I'm a very strong person, I felt like I had a fever. Probably my subconsciousness, that understood how serious and terrifying this could be for me, was reacting.

Consciously I tried to reject the possibility of a relapse.

CA 19-9 is a good marker for pancreatic cancer. The pancreas is a common site for a relapse following colorectal cancer.

Pancreatic cancer is asymptomatic, usually the patient feels nothing unusual.

When detected at a late stage, there is a four to five percent 5-year survival rate.

What an outlook...

If it had actually been the case, it would have ruined my theory about sports and good nutrition being the cure for all illnesses!

At this point, at least until the tests were repeated, I had acquired a new status: **"suspected of a cancer relapse"**...

CHAPTER 18

....

Mind Over Matter

The quote below is attributed to Marilyn Monroe:

"The sky is not the limit. Our mind is."

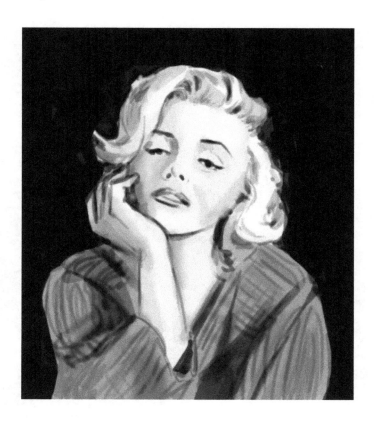

Everything originates in the mind.

There are moments of doubt, and whether I continue or not, go for it and fight or give up, depends only on my determination.

Determination is ruled by the mind.

I owe all my sport achievement to the mind first.

Pursuing training is the result of the mind's decision.

CHAPTER 19
••••••••••••••••••
Meditation

Our well-being is built on four pillars: physical activity, proper nutrition, social life (friends, family, and community) and mental or spiritual attitude.

Most people believe in God and that can definitely be helpful, when they are true believers and their faith is deep and strong.

For many it is just habit, something shallow, not having much significant impact on their lives.

In modern times, in the Western World, many ancient Eastern techniques have been introduced that are greatly contributing to the quality of life of many people.

I'm one of these.

I learned Transcendental Meditation (TM), as taught by Maharishi Mahesh Yogi, when I was 27 and it has changed my life.

It has given me greater peace of mind, short periods of effective rest during the afternoon, that enable me to perform well for the rest of the day, a "shrink" in times of crisis and a great tool for dealing with stressful situations.

It has also opened for me a window into the spiritual world.

Before I started meditating using TM, being a mathematician,

I never gave much thought to such terms as awareness, consciousness or of being in a "place" beyond one's thoughts.

Since then I have also tried Vipassana and other techniques, but I find that for me TM is the simplest, the easiest and most effective. Simple things work the best.

I warmly recommend everybody to try this or another technique.

Without some spirituality in our life, we are not living life to its fullness and are missing an important aspect of life.

How does it work?!

Actually, it's quite simple.

First of all, we need to set aside some time. At least 20 minutes. 25 is better. For me it sometimes reaches to half an hour or even a bit longer.

But sometimes I may have only 10 minutes, and still I get results.

But this is after many years of meditation, so now it is enough for me to simply close my eyes, and I'm "there."

If there is something "urgent" on the table, it's better to finish with that first before meditating, otherwise you may find yourself thinking about it and that can be disturbing.

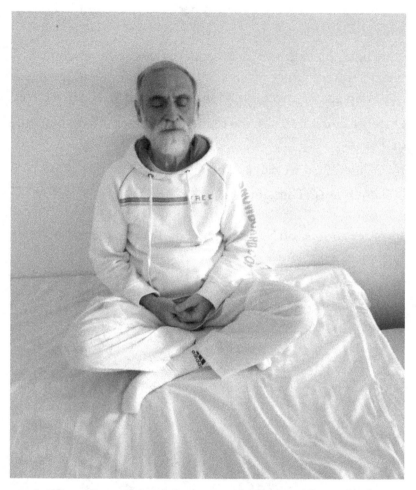

At Bijauri International Campus at the Brahmasthan of India.

The second thing is to sit comfortably, not necessarily in a perfect lotus position. For most people it is enough to just cross your legs together.

A comfortable chair will suffice.

It is better to not be lying down because you might fall asleep and miss the effect.

Dim light, or darkness is also good, but the most important thing is to keep your eyes shut. Vision is responsible for most of our brain activity, accounting for as much as 70 to 80 percent.

Once we close our eyes, the brain immediately drops into second gear.

If it's quiet, then we can go down to first gear.

What remains? Thoughts.

In order to "get rid" of thoughts, in Transcendental Meditation, we use a mantra.

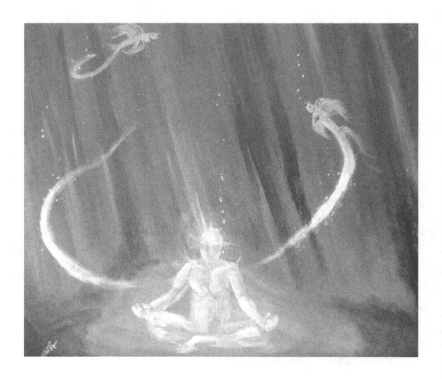

Your personal mantra is your intimate secret. It's a sound that you receive from your TM teacher that you must not disclose to anyone.

You also never say it aloud, except repeating it once or twice at the "initiation" lesson.

Therefore, for your mind, it is associated with inner quiet, and it brings you there, when you mentally repeat it to yourself.

In practice, you never completely get rid of your thoughts. Usually only for brief moments.

So, it is like a kind of inner game: mantra-mantra-thoughts-thoughts-thoughts-back-to-mantra etc.

But it definitely has an effect. There are a vast number of impressive testimonies.

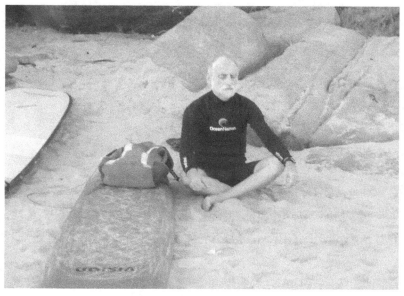

Meditation before surfing in Arugam Bay, Sri Lanka

The key steps are:

Decide to try

Try

Keep going, don't give up if it doesn't work for you from the first moment. It will come. I promise.

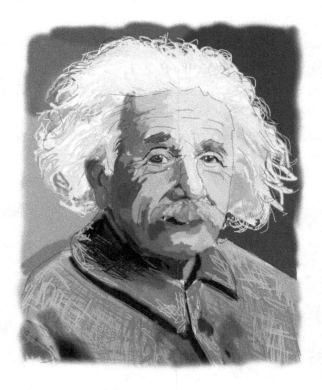

The most beautiful thing we can experience is the mysterious. It is the source of all true art and science." **Albert Einstein**

For sport performance and achievement, it is crucial to train regularly, but is also extremely important to know when to take a break and to occasionally rest.

Once or twice a year, I go for a few days to a retreat to meditate with others.

As opposed to the relatively short meditations that I do at home, twice a day, around a half hour each, during the retreat we meditate much more.

The daily schedule is comprised of several "rounds" in the morning and afternoon, each includes some yoga exercises, some breathing techniques, meditating, resting and then repeating.

We do it in a group, which creates a unique group effect. Hard to explain, but everybody feels it.

During that time, no television, no news, only some advanced video lectures by Maharishi Mahesh Yogi.

At the end of the summer, I went for a 4-day retreat on the campus of the Hebrew University in Jerusalem, where I had studied for my Bachelor of Science and Master of Science degrees, so it was also a bit nostalgic for me.

Following these four days, I felt very rejuvenated, with lots of energy.

Heading toward the triathlon season and my first half marathon, it was like the calm before the storm.

I go for such 3 to 4 day retreats from time to time, but at least once a year.

Summary

- **Our well-being is built on four pillars: physical activity, proper nutrition, social life (friends, family, community) and mental or spiritual attitude.**
- Meditation opens to us a window to the spiritual world
- It provides for greater peace of mind
- 20 minutes of mediation in the afternoon provides a short but effective rest, enabling us to perform well for the rest of the day
- A "shrink" in crisis times – always available
- A great tool when dealing with stressful situations.

CHAPTER 20

A Second Chance

After the 4 days of meditation and no physical activity, I repeated the tests – both markers dropped. Not a lot: CA 19-9 by 8 percent and CEA by 2 percent.

But for me it was enough.

My reasoning was that if I was experiencing a real come back of the cancer, they would have continued to increase.

The turn in direction, following the break, confirmed for me that the previous increase had been caused by my intensive sport activity.

But if it had not been for my initiative to seek another explanation for the rise of the markers and for the help of Tehilla and other friends, I could have repeated the tests following a 17K or an even longer run, and probably gotten even worse results.

That would have led to many more unnecessary tests, to increased psychological pressure and even worse.

This is a good example of why we should always be heavily involved in everything that relates to us, and to not rely with closed eyes on our doctors or on others.

CHAPTER 21

•••••••••••••••••

Another Twist in the Plot

I planned to run my first half-marathon on November 1st 2019, in Haifa. It is a relatively easy run, no hills to climb, and I knew the track quite well.

I wanted to sign-up, but the registration wasn't open yet.

Incidentally, I saw that another half-marathon was planned for the same date – The Galilee half-marathon.

Weird. Two half-marathons on the same day, less then 50km distance between them.

I began checking online and came across a short message saying that the Haifa Half-Marathon was being canceled due to budget cuts.

The Galilee half-marathon on the one hand, was the opposite of the Haifa Half-Marathon – climbing and more climbing.

I knew the first uphill from being in the Achziv Triathlon, when I covered it by bike. It was really quite difficult.

But my mind was already "wired" for running on November 1st.

My friend Habib, a marathon runner, confirmed that it was challenging and recommended that I simply try it out.

Great idea, thanks Habib!

The next day I drove to Achziv and tried running the first uphill and back.

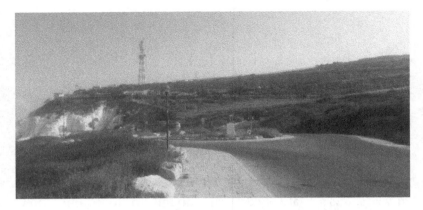

In this photo we can see the first uphill, which continues eastward (right side of photo).

It was really tough and I ran it very slow. But I did it.

It was only 13 kilometers, but it took me one hour and forty minutes, my slowest run ever.

In summary: a very nice landscape, would be a pleasure to run there, difficult, but possible.

I made a quick decision and signed up for this half-marathon!

The photo below shows a close-up of the first hill.

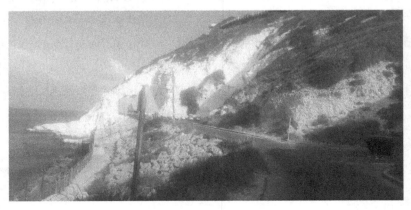

CHAPTER 22
•••••••••••••••••
Running an 18K Run for the First Time!

September 4th. My first 18K!

Really not easy…

Various parts of my body seemed to wake up and start complaining and making demands.

Some of my pains left as quickly as they arrived while others of varying intensity decided to stay.

An interesting process of getting to know one's body…

I liked the second part of the run better. The beginning is always more difficult, the brain probably needs time to understand what I am demanding of it and of my body…

And there are always fears and doubts, just what pains will I be experiencing this time…?

In the past, I would finish each run with a sprint, I really enjoyed it. I like speed.

But now, when the goal is to cover greater and greater distances, I prefer to slow down at the finish to take it easy.

The idea is to not feel completely exhausted at the end but still able to run.

The logic behind this is as follows: I could run that distance and I wasn't exhausted at the end. Therefore, I can run even more!

Next time adding 500 meters, or even more, shouldn't be an issue!

So far it has worked.

In mathematics it's called coming to a conclusion by induction.

According to this math logic, I can run forever. ☺

We will see.

The 18K run took me more than two hours, at an average pace of 6:52 minutes per kilometer.

My average heart rate was 148 beats per minute and maximum heart rate was 171bpm.

My cadence was very slow, only 154 steps per minute.

All in all, a reasonable performance.

CHAPTER 23
••••••••••••••••
Giving-up LSD and Running Faster

During July and August my priority was to extend the distance of each of my runs as I headed toward my first half-marathon on November 1ˢᵗ.

In September I participated in two short races and a triathlon, and gave up distance running.

The first race was the Haifa Night Run, a 10K run that took place on September 12ᵗʰ.

The advantage of the night run was that the heat was more bearable, although the humidity was still very high.

After all of the LSD (Long-Slow-Distance) runs I had experienced, I was full of energy and able to begin the first kilometer with an impressive pace of four minutes and forty-four seconds! My best time ever!

The second kilometer was also very good – 5:11, so I completed the first two kilometers at an average pace of less than 5 minutes per kilometer!

But then the lace of my left shoe came loose. I lost a half minute while tying it. But, even more important, taking that break took me out of my fast pace.

I tried to recover, but then, the second lace came undone…

That was just too much…

Eventually I finished with 54:45, not bad, but I could have done better.

The good news was: I experienced almost no pain in the knee and only a level-3 pain in the left forefeet. Definitely bearable.

The second race was 9 days later, on September 21st and it was my first 10K field run. I enjoyed running in the fields at sunrise, but it is more difficult – the legs don't get that hard road "rebound "when your feet hit the surface and most of the time they just "sink" softly into the ground, requiring much more energy for each stride.

My time wasn't good, 62 minutes, but I enjoyed this new experience.

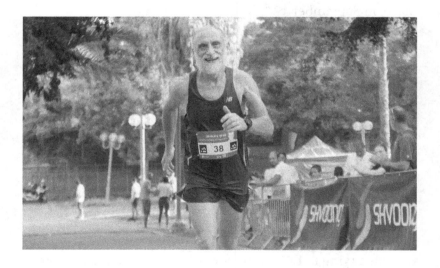

An unexpected outcome of the run was a severe chaffing on both legs.

This had never happened to me before, despite the fact that I am always wet with sweat.

I tried various ointments, but nothing helped and the next few days I couldn't run.

All in all, I had only six day before the triathlon to find a solution.

Eventually tea-tree oil, mixed with olive oil, applied three times a day, solved the problem!

CHAPTER 24

•••••••••••••••••••

The Triathlon Season

September 27th – Netanya Triathlon

A year had passed since my last triathlon, which was followed by the rehabilitation from the partial tear of my left knee patellar tendon.

And I'm a year older, at least biologically...

I'm excited, almost like I was the first time.

I don't take for granted my returning at age sixty-eight and a half, to again compete in a triathlon, with full Olympic distances:

1.5 kilometers swimming in the sea

40 kilometers by bike

10 kilometers run

I like the atmosphere before the event, which begins in the early morning.

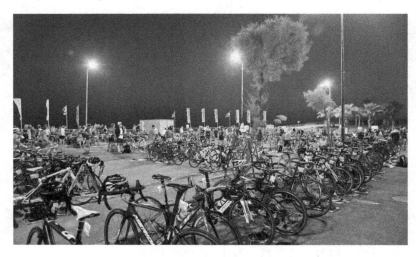

It started with a "mini-drama"; at the beginning of the swim I lost my identity chip! It was swept from my leg and disappeared in the sea.

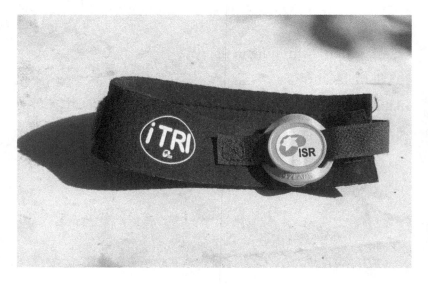

The chip at the beginning of the swim.

Luckily, I found it, but took me time to fix it and when eventually I was ready to go, everybody was already far ahead of me.

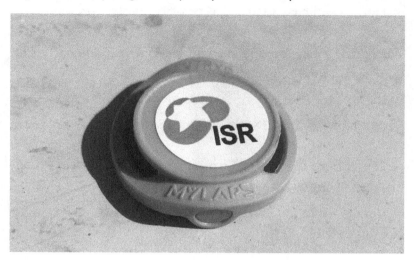

I found myself swimming alone, which is harder psychologically and more difficult technically. I had to raise my head frequently to navigate, instead of just relaying on the legs of the swimmer in front of me.

It was a long swim, it felt like it would never end. At the end the Garmin (my sport watch and best buddy) showed that I had swum 2,250 meters, which is fifty percent longer than the Olympic distance!

After the competition, the organizers admitted that the distance had been 2 kilometers instead of the required 1.5, because the buoys had drifted out with the current...

The other 250 meters I added because I had failed to swim in a straight line and had deviated from one side to the other, especially when returning to shore, I had been blinded by the sun.

I concluded that it is important to swim straight– the shortest distance. I will have to give this priority and to work on it.

The biking was good; my average speed was 26 kilometers an hour with a total time of an hour and half.

Because of the heat, the run was reduced to 5 kilometers.

I eventually finished it with 3:03, still a reasonable time.

At the closing ceremony I was surprised when I was recognized as #1 in my category.

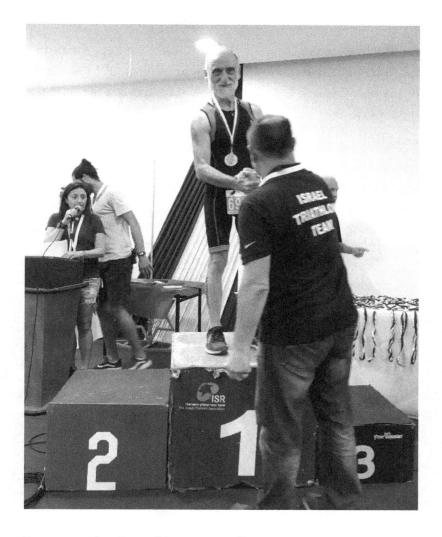

It appears that I was "the category"...

I had planned to take three days off, but after only a one day break, I was already missing the morning activity, so on the second day I went for a swim in the sea - 1.5 kilometers. On the third day I took a short 5K run and on the fourth day I swam for 2 kilometers in the swimming pool.

But my body was telling me that I should have kept the promise to rest and after being in the swimming pool I got a pain in my chest, which lasted the whole day, and left me only the next morning.

Next time I'll keep my promise.

CHAPTER 25
• • • • • • • • • • • • • • • • • •
The Day of the Race, Before and After

There are no two identical races!

Since we are not robots and a run is not carried out under "sterile" experimental conditions, everything influences everything and **has an impact on us; how we run, how we feel, how we perform.**

The event begins the day before. It is the day we eat more complex carbohydrates to build up the stores of glycogen in the muscles.

It is a rest day. Actually, some runners rest even two or three days before the race.

Such a prolonged rest creates a "hunger to run, "and we have more energy, both physically and mentally.

Scan your body for tightened muscles. Massage them with a foot treatment cream or the arnica massaging oil.

One last thing; go to sleep early, so you can wake-up early, but still have enough sleep. Usually, at least six hours.

On race day I wake up early. At least an hour before I intend to leave home. A shower is great, have a snack and take care of all of your other physiological needs.

Also, it is good to be at the race site a bit early. I usually arrive at least a half hour before the race begins. To familiarize myself with the surroundings, have time to perform pre-**run warm-up exercises**, even to run a few minutes, take care of any other physiological needs and have a last opportunity for fueling: I will usually take an energy gel or a date, depending on how I feel.

There are also environmental factors to consider; like the weather and the course that is to be run.

Even on a really cold day, after running a few minutes you will begin to sweat. So as to not suffer too much during the half hour before the run and during the first five to ten minutes of the run, it is a good idea to have something light to put on like a light jacket or sweatshirt, that you can later take off and throw to the side after you have warmed up, that will hopefully still be there when you return to pick it up.

Rain is a major factor, especially if you are running through fields since this can result in muddy puddles that will determine which shoes should be worn.

I like when the rain begins during the race, not at the beginning, as it is excellent for cooling you off.

After the run.

First, the most important thing is to to maintain the balance of your bodily fluids. This is important starting from the moment that you complete your run and throughout at least the following half day.

Eating is less important, but it is good to maintain your blood sugar level, and especially to avoid too sharp of a drop in sugar.

Regarding protein, I'm not a strong believer in the need for a lot of protein. From 10 to 20 grams during the first two to three hours following the race should be quite sufficient.

We do not lose a lot of protein during a run, and building muscles is a slow process.

What we definitely lose during the race are electrolytes, which are lost through sweating.

I take one electrolyte tablet for each hour of running.

Another crucial thing we should never compromise on is loosening the muscles following the run. For at least 10 minutes. 15 minutes is better.

If you can afford it, you should have a professional massage, with emphasize on the tight muscles, you will enjoy your body more, suffer less, and be better prepared for the next run.

After taking care of these physiological needs, take some time to review the event, recall your feelings, sum up what you experienced, draw conclusions, have fun!

CHAPTER 26
•••••••••••••••••••
Running, Swimming and Cycling

October 4th – Hever 15K Run.

In competitive running the adrenaline is pumping and your performance improves. Therefore, I gave up my weekly long run on Wednesday, took a 2-day break to accumulate more energy and glycogen in my body and on Friday at 6:30 AM began my 15 kilometer "journey," together with another thousand runners.

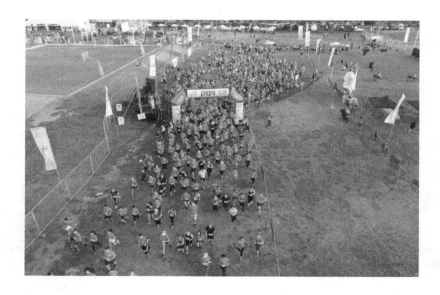

It was a good run, I felt light and full of energy.

The weather was good, not too hot yet in these early morning hours. I like to run in the beautiful Hayarkon Park in Tel Aviv.

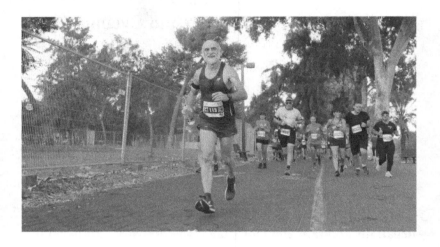

My time was 1:29:32 pace 6:04. I hope I will be able to run the half marathon four weeks from today, at this pace.

My average HR was 162, maximum rate 171, reasonable.

October 16th – 18K run for the second time

The last long run before the half-marathon. Checking my gear, especially the shoes – Altra Paradigm 4.5. They are a bit heavy, but provide the best protection for my left forefoot, a key concern for me in a long run.

It took me 2 hours and 11 minutes, at a pace of 7:15min/km. Very slow, but I did it easily. Average HR was only 142 and maximum 162.

This is my benchmark – in a worst case scenario the half

marathon will take me two hours and 40 minutes.

That's it, I'm ready!

Gan-Shmuel Triathlon - October 26th

The week before the race I participate in another triathlon. This time a sprint-distance triathlon – only half the distance of the Olympic-distance triathlon: 750 meters swimming, 20 kilometers on the bike and a short 5K run.

I was especially happy with my swimming time, 23 minutes, at 3:02 minutes per 100 meters.

It went very smoothly and I finished in 1:44. I saw on the display that I had finished third in my age category so I went to rest before the ceremony.

I returned later to receive my medal, but when the time came for the ceremony, another name was called!

I was quite shocked, but after checking it appeared that my name didn't appear on the list at all.

It took me two days and several e-mails to find out what had happened, but eventually the answer came that I had been disqualified!

One time point was missing in my run.

I was very upset and submitted an appeal. I asked them which time point were they referring to in such a short 5K run?!

It took another week, until I received a confirmation that the appeal was received.

However, up until the time of writing I have still not received a formal answer.

Unofficially, I was told that most probably it was a mistake.

CHAPTER 27
....
The Secrets of my Body

Tomorrow I'll run my first half marathon. I'm in good physical condition and have trained for this event almost half a year.

But the preparations are never perfect. The maximum distance I have run so far is 18 kilometers. The additional three kilometers that I will have to run in the half marathon can be quite challenging. Also, I haven't trained much up hills, and the route is quite steep in at least two parts of the race.

The weather forecast is okay, a chilly morning, when we start the race at 6:30am. But, also a light rain, which may be not so pleasant, at least at the beginning, when I am not yet sweating.

I am feeling the excitement.

I'm curious about myself; how will I do? How will it feel?!

I believe that on a good day I can run 21 kilometers in two hours, but a pain in the knee or the forefoot, could force me to slow down.

Also, there are the up-hill climbs.

So it might be as much as two and a half hours, or even more.

Although I know my body quite well, what I will experience on this long run is quite unpredictable.

And maybe that's the beauty of it?!

I will definitely know my body better after the race is completed.

Two hours alone with my thoughts will also give me the opportunity to get inside of myself. I may have a few thoughts or possibly no thoughts...

But above all; what will be the condition of the route? It's supposed to be hilly and beautiful.

I am already acquainted with the first 6 kilometers and like them (except for the uphill part...), but the other 15 kilometers?!

Following the uphills there must also be downhills. How fast will I descend?! It is possible to make large strides when running downhill. But it can also be quite dangerous. Large strides are a major source of injuries, and in my case, the right knee may really not like it...

I enjoy the excitement of not knowing, of depending on myself alone.

The Galilee half marathon is known for its beautiful landscape, I'm looking forward to it!

CHAPTER 28
·················
My First Half-Marathon

November 1st 2019.

On the morning of the day of the race day I awake before 3 AM and before the two alarm clocks that I have set for 3:15 AM.

I have a 40 minute drive ahead of me and the roads are scheduled to close at 6 AM.

I have been preparing and training for this event for 6 months and I don't want to take any risks, so the plan is to leave at 4:30.

I take a shower, have my morning tea and by 4 AM I am ready to leave.

I remember the cold early morning air, actually still night air, so I take an inexpensive light coat to wear during the time before the race begins and maybe even for the first kilometer, which I will then toss to the side of the road.

By 5 AM I am at Achziv National Park, north of Haifa, where the event is to take place and I'm not the first...

I do a lot of stretching and warming-up, eat a date, and shortly before the race also take an energy gel.

At 6:30 it is still quite cold, but I decide not to use the coat.

The beginning of the race goes well. I finish the first three kilometers in less than 18 minutes, at a pace of 5:58/km and finish in the middle of the group of 230 runners.

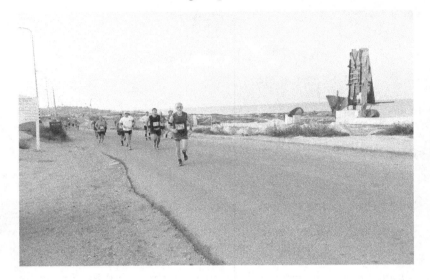

But my heart rate climbs and exceeds 160 bpm, my lactic threshold. I am thinking about the 18 kilometers still ahead of me and slow down a bit, running at 6:30/km.

I have my first "meal" – a date.

After 6 more kilometers the climb begins. It's not too bad. During the beginning I manage to stay at 7min/km, but soon have to switch to a really slow pace of 10 minutes/km, almost walking.

Luckily the climb isn't very long and costs me only 3 to 4 additional minutes.

Many runners pass me, and I think I have fallen back to being among the last 20 or so.

But the uphill climb is followed by the downhill descent and I manage to pick up speed.

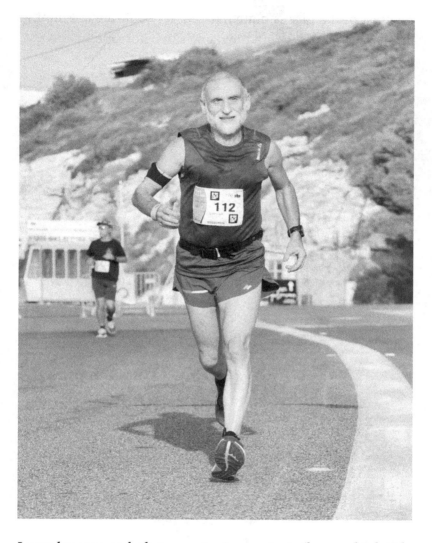

I note by my watch that my pace is now 4min/km, and I decide to slow down, to avoid the risk of additional injury.

I am catching up to the group of runners in front of me.

The rest of the race is quite flat and very enjoyable. Running through green fields with the rising sun before me.

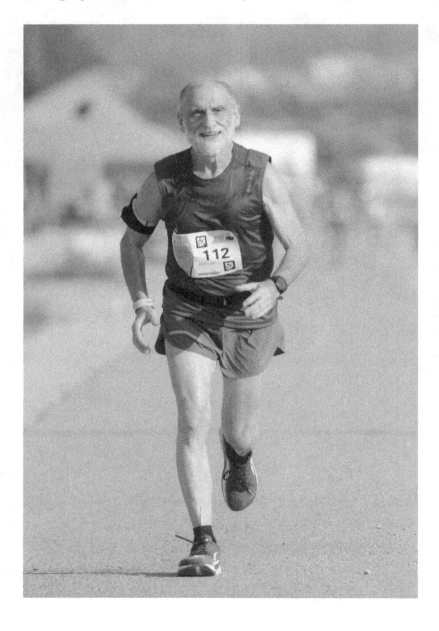

I was passing many runners.

I approach a runner in front of me, then switch into "high gear" for a minute or two and pass him.

I check out my body, nothing is hurting!

WOW, even the knee feels alright.

I am completely focused on moving correctly, not making any mistakes.

After 12 kilometers I have a second "meal" – this time a caffeine gel. It is claimed by some that caffeine catalyzes the absorption of glucose, so why not.

The weather is perfect, so is the air. As I pass a runner I greet him or her with a "Good morning, or How are you?"

I pass the 18 kilometer marker, this is the longest distance I have ever run in a race and I am feeling good.

My average pace is 6:30/km, a bit slow. I know I can run faster, but don't want to push myself too hard.

For me, the main goal of this race is to finish, to prove to myself that I indeed am able to run a half marathon!

I am only 3 kilometers from achieving that goal.

I push myself a little but mostly just enjoy the run.

Eventually, the distance was 400 meters longer and I ran 21.52km.

It has taken me two hours, 18 minutes and 18 seconds, at an average pace of 6:26minutes/km. Less than two and a half hours, but more than my ultimate goal of two hours.

I am happy!

I have just finished my first half marathon and feel fabulous. I'm not at all exhausted. In fact, I feel that I could keep on running!

I am experiencing great feelings of satisfaction and a rush of endorphins.

Endorphins (contracted from "endogenous morphines") are endogenous opioid hormones.

They are produced by the central nervous system and the pituitary gland.

The term "endorphins" implies a pharmacological activity consisting of two parts: endo- and -orphin; these are short forms of the words endogenous and morphine, intended to mean "a morphine-like substance originating from within the body."

The principal function of endorphins is to inhibit the communication of pain signals; but they may also produce a feeling of euphoria very similar to that produced by other opioids.

That's what I was feeling; no pain and mild euphoria.

The following day

The day after, I awake with sore quads.

The full name for quads is quadriceps femoris - a large muscle group that includes the four prevailing muscles on the front of the thigh.

It is the great extensor muscle of the knee, forming a large fleshy mass which covers the front and sides of the femur. The name derives from Latin four-headed muscle of the femur.

I recall the term DOMS, which I have come across in my past readings.

DOMS *(Delayed-Onset Muscle Soreness) is muscle pain that begins* **a day or two after a workout.** *You don't feel DOMS during a workout.*

Pain felt during or immediately after a workout is a different kind of muscle soreness. It's called acute muscle soreness.

Acute muscle soreness is that burning sensation we feel in a muscle during a workout due to a quick buildup of lactic acid. It usually disappears as soon as, or shortly after we stop exercising.

DOMS symptoms typically occur between 12 and 24 hours after a workout. The pain tends to peak about one to three days after the workout, and then begins to ease up.

Symptoms of DOMS to watch out for include:
- muscles that feel tender to the touch.
- reduced range of motion due to pain and stiffness when moving.
- swelling in the affected muscles.
- muscle fatigue.

My quads felt tender when I touched them, range of motion was reduced because of the pain and stiffness when moving – it was DOMS!

High-intensity exercise can cause tiny, microscopic tears in our muscle fibers. Our body responds to this damage by increasing inflammation, which may lead to DOMS in the muscles.

Pretty much any high-intensity exercise can cause DOMS, but one kind in particular, known as eccentric exercise, often triggers it. Eccentric exercises cause us to tense a muscle at the same time we lengthen it.

In my case **it was for sure, the downhill running.**

To ease sore, stiff muscles, it is recommended to keep moving.

We might be tempted to rest and avoid all exercise and movement when DOMS strikes, but unless it's severe, hitting the couch for the day may only worsen the pain and stiffness, not ease it.

To keep muscles moving, you might try practicing a mild form of yoga or do some low to moderate-intensity walking, cycling, or swimming.

Time is the only treatment for DOMS, but we can also take steps to ease the pain and stiffness while we wait for our muscles to repair themselves.

Some findings suggest the following treatments and self-care steps may help lessen the discomfort.

- Massaging during the 48 hours following workout seems to work best. To massage our muscles, we apply some oil or lotion to the affected area and knead, squeeze, and gently shake the muscles.

- Using a foam roller right after a workout may also help head off a bad case of DOMS.

- Topical analgesics, products meant to help relieve pain. Especially those **with arnica** may help ease the pain of DOMS.

- Cold bath; a 10 to 15-minute full-body immersion in a cold-water bath (50–59°F or 10–15°C) lessens the degree of DOMS.

- Warm baths may be helpful too.

I tried some massaging with arnica, working out on my stationary exercise bike at home and a cold bath, and the DOMS decreased quickly.

CHAPTER 29
....
The Beauty of the Freedom to Make Decisions

I have had several sessions with some great coaches and learned from each one.

But on a daily basis I train by myself.

I have plans: long-term, mid-term and some only for the next day.

But I love having the freedom to change my plans, to change them according to the whisper of my intuition, or in adjustment to various unexpected constrains, changes in the weather or simply a sudden desire to go to the beach or to just take a run.

I love my independence and ability to make decisions.

During my career, I have been fortunate to serve in several positions, where I was allowed to act independently: such as project manager, military attaché (no boss at all…) and CEO and chairman of the board of several start-up companies. Well, there was always the Board of Directors to contend with, but on daily basis. I was allowed to act quite independently.

In this context I would like to remind you of a well-known story:

King Arthur was very sick.

The best doctors of the kingdom were unable to cure him and declared that there was no remedy for his illness.

Eventually an old sage offered a solution: there is a witch who can cure any disease.

Since this was the last option, Lancelot, King Arthur's best knight went to the witch.

She agreed to cure King Arthur.

Lancelot was very happy.

"But on one condition," she added, "you will have to marry me."

WOW! the witch was quite old and ugly, while Lancelot was a very handsome young man.

But he was ready to sacrifice everything for his King.

When King Arthur heard of the witch's demand, he said: "No way, you will not sacrifice yourself."

But Lancelot was determined and told the witch: "OK, if you cure the King, I'll marry you."

The witch smiled.

The next day, the king woke up feeling very well and happy.

Lancelot, a man of honor, went to the witch to set up the wedding.

She told Lancelot: I have some good news for you: I can be the witch as you see me now, but I can also be young and beautiful. You have the choice:

Have me young and beautiful during the day, so you can be proud of your new wife, but old and ugly at night.

Or, the opposite, I'll be old and ugly witch during the day, but at nights you will enjoy being with a young beauty.

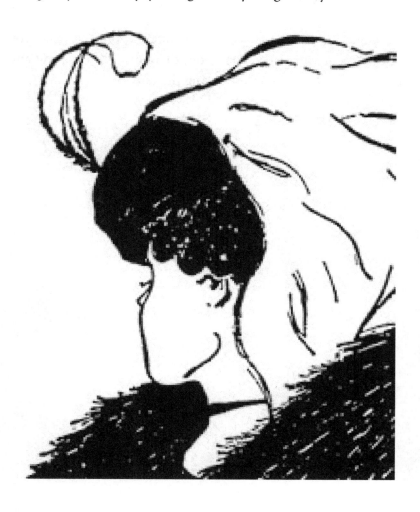

This was a really tough choice.

Eventually Lancelot told the witch: "Thanks for giving me these two options, but I will leave the decision to you."

The witch was very happy! Lancelot, the famous knight, was letting her decide!

In reply she announced: "I very much appreciate that you are letting me make this decision, therefore I'll be young and beautiful both at night and during the day!"

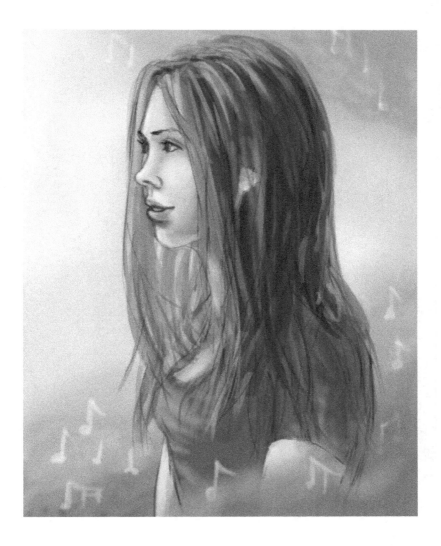

Conclusion: It is good to have the freedom to make decisions. But it is nice also for others. Therefore, we should delegate some of our responsibilities to others; our kids, partner, friends, employees. Then, they too, will enjoy this freedom and the outcome might be surprisingly and unexpectedly good.

CHAPTER 30

····················

The Evolution of My Master Plan

I decided to decrease the number of easier competitive races (10k) and Sprint Triathlons, and to give priority to more endurance type events: By competing in races of 15K or longer and Olympic triathlons.

At this stage, the overhead of each event and the time (the break-day before and the break-day after), and my deviating from my "Master Plan, "was not worth the outcome."

In November I participated in only one competitive race – the Eyal 15K Run.

It had several uphill portions and almost half of it was along dirt roads through fields. All in all, quite tough.

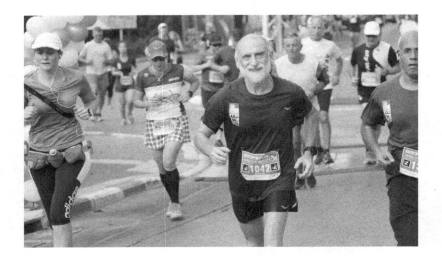

At one point we were running along the security fence of the Army's Unit 8200, in which I served for over 17 years.

Seeing the fence caused strong nostalgic feelings to arise in me making the race even more unique and exciting, and my motivation was higher than ever.

Along the fence, instead of soldiers, an R2D2-like robot was sliding back and forth on its rail.

But within the base, the antennas on the towers looked just the same.

My average pace was 6:18/km and I finished in one hour and thirty three minutes, not a great time, but still ahead of hundreds of much younger runners.

I mentioned Unit 8200. Unit 8200 is the SIGINT (Signal Intelligence) division of Israeli Intelligence. Once it used to be quite secret, but in recent years it has become famous for its extraordinary performance, innovations and high standard of quality. Numerous world-class start-ups, some of which have evolved into large multi-national enterprises, some acquired by giant corporations, were founded by alumni of that unit. A good example is CheckPoint, which invented and brought to the world the firewall.

The book *"Spies, Inc.: Business Innovation from Israel's Masters of Espionage"* written by former TIME magazine and monthly magazine Business 2.0, journalist Stacy Perman, allows a glimpse into what the special unit is all about. Perman writes: *"The most highly successful innovation machine in the world. A little known classified high-tech unit in Israeli Intelligence known as 8-200. Its charter is to develop technologies and solutions, customized and suited to the unique challenges of fighting terrorism and endless war."*

At the same time I changed my weekly routine:

I'm still running three times a week, but I have signed-up for a gym membership and have added 45 minutes in their fitness room twice a week, followed by one hour of swimming.

In the gym I work on the muscles which are receiving less attention from my aerobic activities: lat pull-downs, leg extensions, triceps extensions, seated row exercises, shoulder presses, glute presses, chest presses, preacher curls and abdominal curls.

Three sets of fifteen repetitions each.

I combine the gym with the swimming pool, mainly because they are located in the same facility, so it saves me time. But also, it is good to swim after any workout, as it is releasing and relaxing.

All in all, it comes to 10 workouts a week: running three times, bike twice, swim twice, gym twice and once a week 45 minutes of TRX or Pilates with a personal coach.

But most of the workouts are not more than an hour, so I never become too tired, or exhausted.

On the other hand, the synergy of the diversified workouts is one of the keys to being in good shape, and to feeling great.

I also signed-up for a ballroom dancing course.

I found it to be a very pleasant physical activity, awakening new areas in my brain.

Until now (68+), I used only to dance spontaneously without any knowledge, and even that, very rarely.

But I had a romantic "craving" for dancing.

Luckily for me, there was a lady who didn't have a partner, and she agreed to give it a try.

She is much younger than I am, a natural dancer who has also danced in the past, while for me it was the first time.

The first lesson was quite a disaster and I was ready to give up.

But both the teacher and my new partner encouraged me to not make a decision after only one lesson.

We extended the trial for another two lessons. I bought a DVD from the teacher teaching beginner's steps, I practiced at home and made significant progress.

Following the successful trial, we decided to continue.

During the first 15 lessons we learned Basic Steps, Paso Doble, Mambo, English Waltz, Square Tango, Padegras, and a sequence dance: Salsa Mexicana.

Sequence dance is a form of dance in which a preset pattern of movements is followed, usually to music which is also predetermined. The big advantage is that the patterns are standard-universal, so it is possible to dance with a partner with whom you are not previously acquainted and in any setting.

We both enjoy it very much, and I think that our teacher enjoys seeing us progress.

CHAPTER 31

Pseudo-Schizophrenia and My Alter-Ego

Schizophrenia does not imply a "split personality," a condition with which it is often confused in the public perception.

Schizophrenia is a mental disorder characterized by abnormal behavior, strange speech and a decreased ability to understand reality.

Other symptoms include false beliefs, unclear or confused thinking, hearing voices that do not exist, reduced social engagement and emotional expression, and lack of motivation. As of 2013, there was no objective test for schizophrenia.

About 0.5 percent of people are affected by schizophrenia during their lifetime.

In 2013, there were an estimated 24 million cases globally.

But I will use here the common perception of a "split personality," to define my mental illness.

I think I suffer from a new kind of mental disease, which I'll call "pseudo-schizophrenia." ☺

When I run on the beach in the morning and see the waves, they look frightening to me, really. Such vast sea power!

Just the other day, I woke up early in the morning and went to go surfing.

I must admit, that until I'm in the water, I'm quite unsettled; the cold water, the strong waves... sometimes jellyfish.

But once I'm on my surfing board, and I feel the sea beneath me, my "alter ego" appears!

I forget my fears and begin paddling and enjoying myself!

From the sea, I see people running on the beach, it looks difficult to me, how far can they possibly run. What about the fatigue?!

But again, the very next day, I myself go out for a run. Before I take my first step I feel cold and am not sure how it will go.

I tell myself: "buddy, you've done this many times!"

I start running, and my alter-ego kicks in, I forgot all of my previous thoughts and begin to run easily, flowingly and almost effortlessly, with great joy and pleasure.

I experience similar feelings before diving and skiing.

When diving, the first "giant step" into the water is frightening.

But once I'm 10 to 15 meters below the surface, the quietude and the view induce calm, and I very much enjoy myself. Pseudo-schizophrenia...

My Alter Ego.

An alter ego (Latin for "other I") is a second self, which is believed to be distinct from a person's normal or true original personality. A person who has an alter ego is said to lead a double life. The term appeared in common usage in the early 19th century when dissociative identity disorder was first described by psychologists.

Cicero coined the term as part of his philosophical construct in First-century Rome, but he described it as "a second self, a trusted friend."

The existence of "another self" was first recognized in the 1730s. Anton Mesmer used hypnosis to reveal the alter ego. These experiments showed a behavior pattern that was distinct from the personality of the individual when he was in the waking state compared with when he was under hypnosis. Another character had developed in the altered state of consciousness but in the same body.

Alter ego is also used to refer to the different behaviors any person may display in certain situations.

In fiction; Dr. Jekyll and Mr. Hyde

The title characters in Robert Louis Stevenson's thriller *The Strange Case of Dr. Jekyll and Mr. Hyde* represents an exploration of the concept that good and evil exist within one person, constantly at war.

Edward Hyde literally represents the doctor's other self, a psychopath who is unrestrained by the conventions of civilized society, and who shares a body with the doctor. The names "Jekyll and Hyde" have since become synonymous with a split personality or an alter ego that becomes capable of overpowering the original self.

Why is this so?!

I believe, the second nature (or maybe the first one) is what we want to do, but are not accustomed to doing.

Or, maybe, we are afraid to leave our comfort zone?!

I didn't start surfing until I was 65 years of age, and wasn't doing any serious running before this time either.

Now, my first ego and my alter ego, have to fight each other and convince one the other, what's right and what's wrong for a 70 year old guy, who feels like he's 17…

Maybe because of his compromised hearing, seventy sounds to him like seventeen… ☺

Or maybe it's a form of self-hypnosis?!

CHAPTER 32

·················

My Second Half Marathon

December 6th – The Valley of Springs

As my second half marathon approaches, I begin decreasing the level of my sport activities.

The main reason being my stores of glycogen.

I learned that it takes me time to replenish the glycogen in my muscles. The pace of building glycogen is very individual and is influenced by one's diet. The more glucose in the blood, the faster the glycogen stores are built. But my diet isn't very sweet…

So, I prefer not to use the cumulated glycogen before the race, and the last two days before the race I enjoy taking it easy.

My feelings before the race. Despite knowing myself and my physical abilities quite well, and having already run one half marathon, I don't really know how well I will do the second time.

According to logic and experience, most probably my pace will be around 6 minutes per kilometer, add a minute at the beginning and 2 to 3 additional minutes for the Bet-Shaan uphill climb. That would make two hours and nine minutes.

Or it could go the opposite way, a minute less at the beginning and an additional 2 to 3 at the end (after all 21 kilometers could cause some tiredness…), so 2:10.

And there is also wishful thinking that maybe I'll outdo myself and achieve my ultimate goal of two hours?!

The drive from my home to the motel at Kibbutz Nir David takes 75 minutes.

It appears that the starting line at Gan HaShlosha National Park "The Garden of the Three" is not very close to where I am staying at the kibbutz.

It begins to rain and heavy rains are forecasted for that afternoon and also on the day of the race.

Before the rains get too hard, I go to check out the race venue and the course.

I met and old man (actually about my age…) and asked him the way.

"You can't go there, there is no way through."

"But I have to get there," I insist.

"The only option is by the main road outside the Kibbutz, but it's more than two kilometers, don't you have a car?!"

Instead of explaining that two kilometers is really not much for one who is planning to run 21.1 kilometers the following day, I change the subject.

"You know, some 50 years ago, when I immigrated from Poland to Israel, I began my 'new life' right here, in this Kibbutz. I was working then in the grapefruit orchard and studying Hebrew. The name of my teacher sounded like Manta, but not Manta. For the past 50 years, I have been trying to reconstruct her name. Maybe you knew her?"

This time his reply was immediate: "Of course, her name was Matla, I married her daughter. She passed away a long time ago..."

Matla! Right, that sounded right! After 50 years...

I thanked the man, and walked toward the main road, while eating the sandwich I had brought from home.

The remembrance of my first Hebrew teacher, 50 years earlier, awakened in me strong feelings of nostalgia.

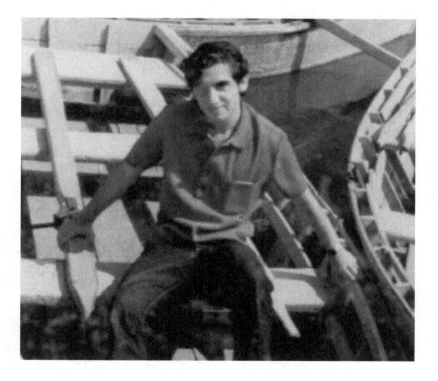

That's how I looked then.

I loved those days!

The guard at the gate also couldn't understand, why was I walking instead of driving a car. Weird people…

It was indeed about 2 kilometers and it took me 20 minutes.

The place had not yet been prepared for tomorrow's race, but there was one clear sign that a public event was about to take place – a long line of chemical toilets… very typical of all races and triathlons…

I walked back another 20 minutes in the rain. By 5 PM I was back in my room, #5, and fell into deep meditation.

Friday, December 6th – the race day.

I slept well and awakened at 5 AM, before either of my two alarm clocks.

I eat a hundred calorie energy bar with my traditional morning green tea and take a shower.

I drive my car to the kibbutz gate, so that I now have to walk only 1.5 kilometers.

It takes me 15 minutes and by 7 AM I am at "The Garden of the Three," Gan HaShlosha National Park.

Three thousand runners are participating in this race, therefore it is quite crowded.

The race is supposed to start at 8:05 AM, so I walk around, probably accumulating at least 3 kilometers before the race even starts – a good warm-up.

I also do a lot of stretching, have one GU gel and one date. I'm ready!

The wait at the starting line always feels long.

Actually, there is a short delay and at 8:09 the mass of three thousand runners begins to move.

The fastest runners are in the front lines while the slowest are in the back, to avoid "collisions," and almost immediately the mass of runners forms into a line. A somewhat thick line, but still a line.

The first 5 kilometers go by quite easily. Probably because of my two-day rest, the accumulated energy which wants to burst out and the build-up accumulated glycogen.

My pace is 5:50 minutes per kilometer and I finish the first 5 kilometers in 29 minutes and am feeling great.

In the next 5 kilometers there is a slight rise leading to a bridge and I slow down a bit. But I still manage to complete the first 10 kilometers in one hour and a few seconds.

I take a gel at the 6th km and eat a date after 10 kilometers.

I also stop at a water station and refill one of the two small bottles I am carrying.

This costs me around two minutes and I finish 15 kilometers in 92 minutes.

The third part of the run was the most pleasant for me, a straight run with no climbs under blue skies, instead of the expected rain.

But at the 16th kilometer we enter the town of Beit-Shean and it is one continuous climb. Not steep, but continuous and long.

By this time my body is feeling a bit tired and the fourth 5 kilometers go quite slowly, at a pace of 7min/km – for a total of 35 minutes and I complete 20 kilometers in two hours and 7 minutes.

I complete the last 1.1 kilometers at a good pace of 6min/km finishing the race in two hours and 14 minutes.

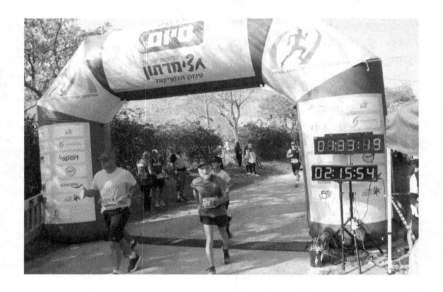

Not exactly as expected but all in all reasonable and four minutes faster than my first half marathon five weeks ago.

As long as I see an improvement I'm satisfied.

I enjoyed the experience very much and the distance.

I finished 1,700[th] out of 3,000, leaving behind me some 1,300 runners, 99 percent of them much younger than me.

And I still wasn't exhausted.

Adding my walks before and after the race, that morning my legs had covered over 25 kilometers and I was feeling great!

Most importantly; I was feeling almost no pain in my knee and left forefoot.

CHAPTER 33

·················

Recovery

The first things that I do following an event are:

- Stretching
- Moving
- Hydrating

Usually, I'm not hungry immediately after the event. That comes later, and even then I do not eat large meals.

I first get some simple sugars like by eating a baguette and then I'll have a Nature Valley Protein bar.

I shower of course, whenever possible.

After the shower, and while the body is fueled with some sugars and is well hydrated, I lie down to rest.

Meanwhile, 2 to 3 hours have passed, the level of endorphins is declining, and I typically fall into a deep sleep.

But usually for not more than an hour.

After about four hours, I'm recovered enough that I am able to perform any of my routine activities, although I do feel the muscles in my legs. This time especially the back of the lower leg is quite stiff and going down the stairs is challenging.

It's also a good time for a more substantial meal, like my BAL meal, sometimes in a more fluid form, like a soup.

To celebrate the event, it's time for a glass of wine or my favorite single malt The Balvenie whisky.

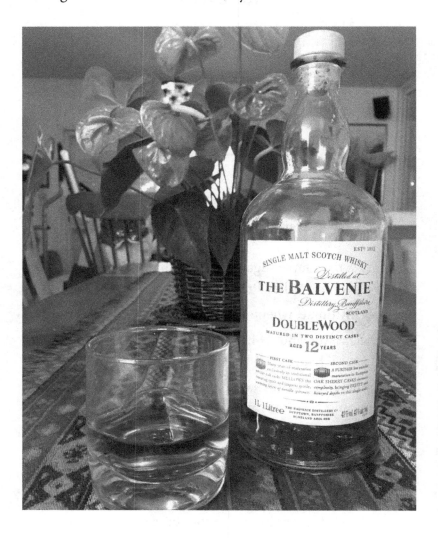

After 48 hours, I would say that I am 90 percent recovered.

On the third day I go for an easy, relaxing swim. I also enjoy a natural water massage in the Jacuzzi and try the sauna.

On the fourth day: back to biking. Fifth day: gym + swimming pool, as usual, and on the sixth day, 120 hours following the half marathon, I start running again, with pleasure.

To summarize: The 6:20 minutes per kilometer pace was not as I had hoped, but the recovery was really fast, after 5 days I'm running again, and ready for the third half marathon four weeks after the second.

Therefore, the overall balancing is good.

CHAPTER 34

·················

In Unity

During our daily 24-hour cycle, we experience three states of consciousness: being awake, asleep and dreaming.

In some Eastern cultures, in ancient India for example, mainly as recorded in the Vedas (Veda means knowledge in Sanskrit), other states of consciousness are described; Transcendental Consciousness, Cosmic Consciousness (CC), God Consciousness (GC) and Unity Consciousness (UC).

When we are awake, we are always aware of something and have many thoughts. When we are in a deep transcendence, we may attain moments that transcend thinking. When we have no thoughts, only then are we aware of pure being only.

This is what happens to me when I meditate, but also many times during long runs.

The more we experience a state of being beyond thoughts, the more higher states of consciousness unfold and develop within us. We see things more clearly and enjoy our daily lives more.

At some point of time in our lives we may attain higher levels of consciousness.

According to the ancient Vedic Scripts there are 7 States of Consciousness:

1. Being awake
2. Sleep
3. Dreaming
4. Transcendental Consciousness (TC) - reaching beyond thoughts, usually during deep meditation.
5. Cosmic Consciousness (CC) - experiencing TC in daily life!
6. God Consciousness (in the Bible there is a beautiful passage – "God is within you.")
7. And ultimately, when you reach a state of full enlightenment– Unity Consciousness (UC). Becoming one with everything!

When I run, I'm more aware of my body. I am able to sense the slightest change or feeling.

I feel my body, observe it as it moves, almost effortlessly, almost by itself. But I also "feel" the road.

My feet are lightly touching the ground, for a fraction of a second, but feeling it.

I feel myself and my body. They are one thing.

This is my interpretation of Unity Consciousness.

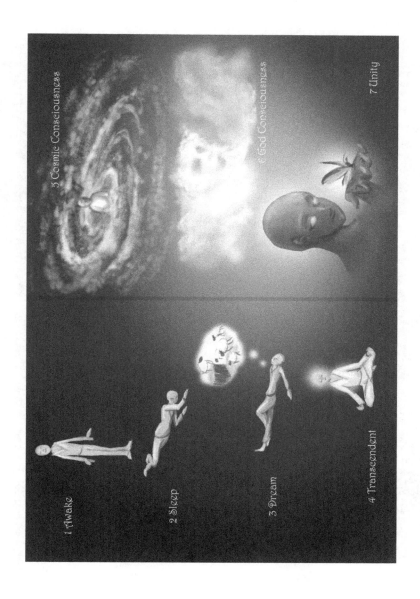

1 Awake
2 Sleep
3 Dream
4 Transcendent
5 Cosmic Consciousness
6 God Consciousness
7 Unity

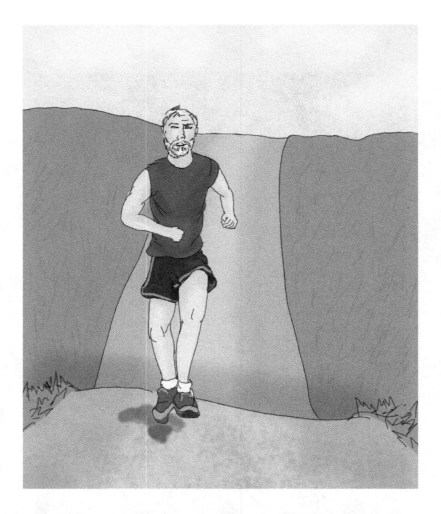

I definitely do not pretend to be in Unity Consciousness, as meant in Eastern teachings.

But when I am in the midst of a long distance run, I enter a kind of transcendent state and am in unity with my path.

In the half marathon my sense of this UNITY becomes stronger than ever.

CHAPTER 35

The Formula

I feel that I have found the formula for staying young and for performing very well on a daily basis, and would like to share this formula with you.

By implementing this formula, we can live practically forever.

I want to claim that biologically the body doesn't have to age, IF WE LIVE CORRECTLY.

You may say, but everyone becomes old, so we have to age.

My claim is, that it doesn't have to be so.

You may not believe me.

But it's true and I'm sure, that after reading this book you will agree with me.

When the cells of our body are replaced by new cells, these cells are created according to the same DNA as the original cells. The DNA doesn't age; when we are young and when we are old, we still have the same DNA.

Actually, the only biological process which changes with time is the shortening of telomers.

A telomere – "end-part" (in Greek telos - end and meros - part), is a region located at each end of a chromosome, which protects its end from deterioration or from fusion with neighboring chromosomes.

Empirical evidence shows that the telomeres associated with each cell's DNA will slightly shorten with each new cell division until they reach a critical length making further cell division impossible.

In 2009 Elizabeth Blackburn, Carol Greider, and Jack Szostak were awarded the Nobel Prize in Physiology or Medicine for the discovery of the way chromosomes are protected by telomeres.

The estimations are that there are between 50 and 75 trillion cells in the body. Each type of cell has its own life span. Red blood cells live for about four months, some white blood cells live very shortly but most live for more than a year. Skin cells live about two or three weeks. Colon cells die after about four days. Sperm cells have a life span of about three days, while brain cells typically last an entire lifetime.

As for heart cells the estimations are that no more than half are replaced during our lifetime.

Even by conservative estimations, most telomers are sufficient to allow for about 150 years of life.

Our mind and body have the capability to deliver a fantastic performance, and to last practically forever.

But they need the right conditions.

In the chapter 19 - "Meditation." I mentioned the four pillars: *physical activity, proper nutrition, social life (friends, family, community) and mental or spiritual attitude.*

In addition to these four pillars there is a very simple but effective practical formula that allows us to get the best from our mind and body, and over a very long period of time.

The formula comprises dividing our daily activity time into three chunks of 5-8 hours each, in addition to three rest periods - the 6 to 7 night hours of sleep along with the addition of two 20 to 30 minute breaks daily for rest or meditation.

Thus, the rest periods, including sleep, will occupy one third of the 24 hour cycle, which may sound like a lot.

Your first reaction might be: "That's a waste of time."

But the point is, that due to this activity-rest-activity-rest cycle formula, our efficiency and efficacy of action multiplies and we get skyrocketing performance!

This formula is both vitalizing and energizing, and will keep us young, healthy and energetic!

As opposed to being exhausted!

Resting is a kind of "investment," but the ROI (return on investment) definitely justifies it.

Just take a look at my bio to see how much I have achieved, despite devoting this much time to sufficient sleep and meditating twice a day.

During these rest periods, the brain can organize itself including its; thoughts, long-term memory; learn from new experiences and plan next steps. A good demonstration of what happens to the brain, when we don't allow it sufficient rest time, is when we are at a conference and after two to three lectures, we begin to feel tired.

With regard to the body, you could view rest breaks as activating a "reset button," allowing the body to "repair" whatever needs to be fixed, build-up proteins, refuel and more.

Another key ingredient in the formula is play!

The following wise saying is attributed to Benjamin Franklin: *"We don't stop playing because we grow old; we grow old because we stop playing."*

Summary:

- The four pillars of a good and happy life are: *physical activity, proper nutrition, social life (friends, family, and community) and mental or spiritual attitude.*

- The formula allowing a long life and exceptional performance comprises dividing our daily activity time into three chunks of 5 to 8 hours each, along with three periods of rest; the six to seven hours of night sleep and two 20-30 minute breaks for rest or meditation.

- This "investment" in sufficient rest brings an unprecedented ROI in terms of longevity and quality of life!

CHAPTER 36

·····················

The Third Half Marathon - Tiberias

As my third half marathon approached, I continued with all of my usual activities: running, swimming, cycling and going to the gym. I believe that my fitness is the result of the synergy of this combination.

Friday, December 20th. Early morning biking.

6:30 AM. At first light I'm out on my bike.

I very soon realize that I am not properly dressed. The temperature is 8 degrees Celsius (a chilly 46F) and the wind is quite strong. The speed of the bike doubles the effect of the wind.

I'm freezing.

But I never compromise on my plans.

"So let it be written, so let it be done" – I like this quote, which I once heard in the movie *"The Ten Commandments,"* spoken by Yul Brinner (playing Pharaoh Rameses II) to his chief architect Baka,

the basic meaning being that once something is set in motion it is final and cannot be altered, so to speak...

I write down my plans, and then realize them, never giving up, if I have decided to do something.

I may compromise on the performance. I'm quite flexible and will make adjustments depending on how I feel on that day, my heart rate etc.

So, I'm freezing, but continue pedaling.

Only after 20 kilometers or so, I begin thawing out…

My mission is accomplished.

Conclusion: next time dress better.

During the coming week I plan to run my last long run, before the half marathon. The preferred date is Wednesday the 25th, 10days before the race. But it's not my final decision yet.

I listen to the weather forecast, "Heavy rains expected for Wednesday."

It may be fun to run in the rain, and I have done it several times. But this time I have other plans for Wednesday and decide on the spot to give up this pleasure and to run the 15k tomorrow - Saturday.

I like to make quick decisions.

I don't have with me the Altra Paradigm 4.5, my long-distance running shoes, and have only the light Escalante with minimum cushioning.

It was a real pleasure; Saturday morning, with no particular plans, not hurrying anywhere.

I start out at 7:30 AM, quite late, so it is already quite warm, 16 degrees Celsius (61F).

Blue skies, no wind, perfect weather.

The first five kilometers go easily, though not very fast, my pace is 6:30 minutes per kilometer.

But also my heart rate has not exceeded 150 bpm.

Five more kilometers, a slight climb. Even slower and the HR reaches 181.

On the positive side, the standard formula that your maximum heart rate should equal 220 bpm minus your age, leads me to the conclusion, that I am age 39.

By the way, when I checked last week what the Garmin calculated for my fitness age, it came to 31!

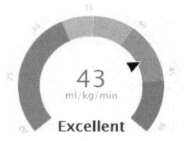

Your VO₂ Max is **43** which is excellent for men ages 60-69. Your fitness age is **31**. That's the **top 10%** for your age and gender.

Garmin tracks everything; all the runs, biking, swimming, fitness room and even just moving.

Between 31 and 39, seems that I'm still in my thirties. ☺

I finish the 15 kilometers in one hour and forty minutes, at a pace of 6:39, quite slow. But enjoy it very much.

After three minutes my heart rate falls below 100, a very encouraging recovery.

I devote the next 17 minutes to stretching and afterward feel that I could take another run.

Tomorrow I will continue as usual, 25 kilometers on the bike.

But this time I will dress warmer.

4 days of meditation

On Wednesday I went for my 4 day meditation retreat in Jerusalem.

In the guest house of the faculty of Humanities we spent many hours in meditation. The morning session lasted some 4 hours and the afternoon three hours. In between were lectures, some mingling and two meals.

Definitely a time of deep rest and of recharging my "batteries" with energy for future use.

I came back on Saturday and during the five days before my third half marathon exercised lightly – so as to not deplete my body's stores of glycogen too much and to maintain my "hunger" for the event.

I arrive in Tiberias Thursday afternoon, pick up my race number – 3791 and the t-shirt.

The walking distance from the hotel to the starting point is less than 10 minutes.

During the whole day it rains and the forecast for the following day, the day of the race is a 70 percent probability of precipitation.

I don't mind running in the rain. It can even be fun, but not at the beginning, when the body hasn't warmed up yet.

On the day of the race I awake at 4 AM, an hour before my two alarm clocks. Plenty of time...

I do some stretching, shower, drink some tea and then more stretching.

Check-out time is quite cruel: 10 AM. I calculate that I will finish the race at around 9:45 + add the 10 minute walk back to the hotel, I'll have just enough time. But what about a shower?!

After some "negotiations," the manager agrees to postpone my check-out time to 10:30. Still, not leaving me much time.

Anyhow, I put most of my stuff in my car, leaving in the room only a change of clothes.

I am happy to see that there are no clouds in the sky! No rain!

But it is really cold, 7-8 degrees Celsius (about 45F).

By 7 AM I am at the starting line, along with some seven thousand other runners. The marathon and half marathon will be run together. Nice.

Of course, after 10.55 kilometers we, (the half marathon runners) will turn back and the marathon runners will continue.

The first 5 kilometers are very pleasant and easy, as usual, 29 minutes, at a pace of 5:48min/km.

I know this part of the race course from the time that I ran my first 10k here, in Tiberias, exactly two years ago.

I am surprised when after some 7 kilometers I reach a climb, although not very steep and not long.

As you already know, I'm not a good uphill runner. I take it easy and finish the first 10 kilometers in 61 minutes, at a pace of 6:06/km. That's not too bad, but below my expectations.

I like the landscape. It is fun to run alongside the very calm Sea of Galilee.

It is over 200 meters below sea level, so the air pressure is high and we get plenty of oxygen.

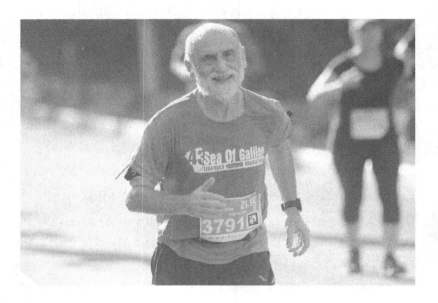

After 12 kilometers I begin feeling some unpleasant sensations in my right knee, and that always causes me to slow down, being afraid of additional injury.

This slowing down results in my finishing the first 15 kilometers in 95 minutes, at a pace of 6:20/km.

The last 6 kilometers aren't fast either and I finish the race in two hours and 16 minutes.

Actually, very similar to my other two half marathons.

The table below summarizes the key parameters in the three runs:

The Event	Dist	Time	Pace	Avg. HBR	Max. HBR	SPM	Stride length
Galilee	21.5	2:18	6:26	163	179	158	98
The Valley	21.2	2:14	6:20	163	183	159	99
Tiberias	21.2	2:16	6:24	159	181	158	99
Average	21.3	2:16	6:23	162	181	158	99

Dist. = the exact race distance. It is supposed to be 21.1km, but many times due to the constrains of the terrain, there are slight variations.

Time - the full run time

Pace – minutes/km

Avg. HBR – the average heart beat rate

Max. HBR – the maximum heart beat rate

SPM – strides per minute

Stride length – the average length of my stride

This was my third half marathon in two months, since the first one on November 1st

Seems that my performance is quite consistent.

The positive side of it is: I can rely on this performance and I think I have earned the title "half marathon runner." ☺

On the less positive side, no signs of improvement.

My conclusions are; my performance is influenced by the fact that I have not been running enough, recently less than 90kms/month and also that whenever I feel any suspicious sensations in my knee, I'm afraid of injury and I slow down.

But I do summarize these three runs with satisfaction.

CHAPTER 37

....

The Second Heart

In my second book: *The Secret of Life*, I dedicate a chapter to the immune system and present arguments as to why physical activity is so important for the best functioning of the immune system and thus our health.

The lymphocytes most of the time are floating in the lymphatic system, comprising a large network of lymphatic vessels that carry a clear fluid called lymph.

Unlike the circulatory system, the lymphatic system does not have its own pump like blood. *The strongest "push" it gets is from the skeletal muscles, when they are active. Then, the lymph reaches all, even the most distant, "corners" of the body, and the immune system is ready to defend us everywhere and anytime. The best health protection prevails.*

Recently I found an additional argument supporting the claim of the contribution of physical activity to the ultimate functioning of the immune system – **the lymph heart!**

A lymph heart is an organ found in lungfish, all amphibians, reptiles and flightless birds and its function is to pump lymph!

These animals aren't very physically active and evolution has equipped them with the lymph heart.

But evolution hasn't provided such a pump to humans, because they were quite physically active.

With the development of civilization; cars, elevators etc. many people are less active and therefore more often ill. Here comes physical activity to bring us back to our nature so that we can live a healthier life.

CHAPTER 38
....
Moments of Joy and Pleasure - the Power of Now!

Following the classic book: *The Power of Now: A Guide to Spiritual Enlightenment* by Eckhart Tolle, whose ideas I am adopting and attempting to fully implement, I try to ask myself several times a day: "Am I enjoying this moment?!"

If the answer is positive, I try to create "more of the same."

If the answer is negative, I ask myself "Why?" and make an effort to correct it.

I wrote down some of the activities I really enjoy:

Meeting family and friends.

The routine of sport activities.

The time after the activity.

Meditating.

Good food.

Good wine or whisky.

Good music.

Dancing.

Playing bridge.

Visiting new places; especially skiing once a year, surfing and diving.

I'm grateful for my good fortune and being able to enjoy all these things.

I think the basis for being able to devote most of my time to these pleasant activities and enjoying them, is being on the right level in the Maslow's hierarchy of needs.

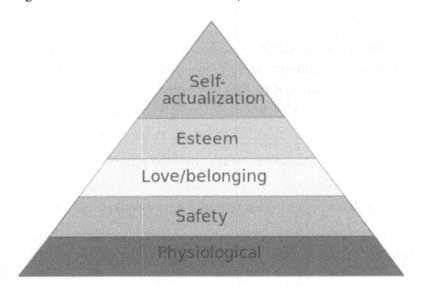

Maslow used the terms "physiological," "safety," "belonging and love," "social needs" or "esteem," and "self-actualization" to describe the pattern through which human motivations generally move. This means that in order for motivation to arise at the next stage, each stage must be first satisfied within the individual themselves.

Everybody can build his or her own list. Each list will be

different, but it helps to become more aware that we all have things and moments that we enjoy, and that we can create more of them.

Usually, it is necessary to first take care of the basic stages in Maslow's pyramid in order to enable us to enjoy life more.

And maybe, it is a form of "self- hypnosis" – telling yourself: I'm going to enjoy myself.

CHAPTER 39
....
"Tough" Times in Seychelles, January 2020

During the last 10 weeks I did a lot of running.

Three half marathons, and I enjoyed them.

But it's time for a break...

Swimming is still my weakest point in the triathlon, so when the opportunity came, I was happy to sign-up for another Open Water training camp, this time in Seychelles.

Most of the swimmers who participated in the Open Water training camp in Maldives in April, nine months ago also signed up for this trip. This should make it even more exciting. I'm looking forward to it!

On January 18th 2020 we landed on Mahe, the largest island in the Seychelles archipelago, containing the city of Victoria, the capital of Seychelles, a country comprising 115 islands with a population of less the 100,000.

On the Sea Bird liveaboard yacht, we were 18 swimmers in nine small two-person cabins with a crew of less than 10, including the captain, the mechanic, the kitchen team and the divemaster.

The sailing time to our first stop was four hours. The ocean was very rough and most of us felt very bad.

For the first three hours I lie on my bed, almost not moving.

But then, I can't stand it anymore, and "give back" to the sea everything I had eaten during the last day or two…

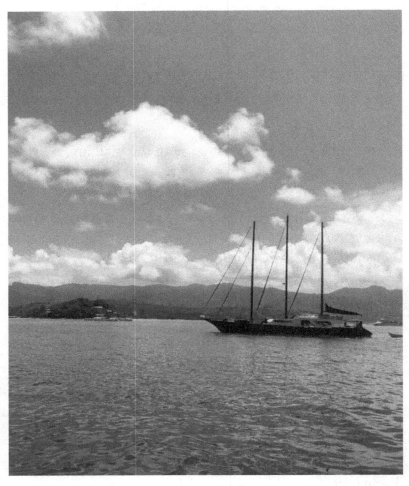

The Sea Bird

During the following days we were moving from island to island, staying at night in a bay, or near an island.

Some of the sailing was rough, but none was as bad as the first day.

Also, probably, the body got used to the waves.

From time to time we would swim to the beach and enjoy the beatiful landscapes of Seychelles.

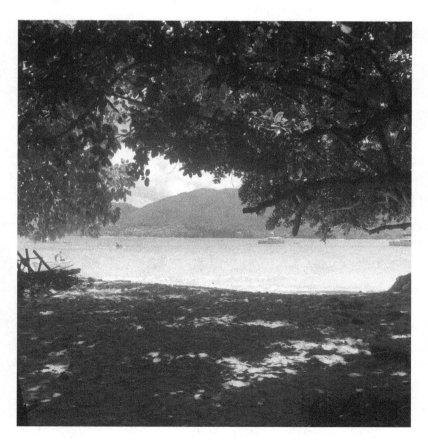

Our routine was swimming up to two hours in the morning, a shorter, technical session in the afternoon and inbetween times, diving.

Swimming in the Indian Ocean wasn't very different from swimming in the Mediterranean Sea. The temperature of the water was 28-29 degrees Celsius (82 to 84F), similar to the air temperature during the day.

But in the evenings it got cooler.

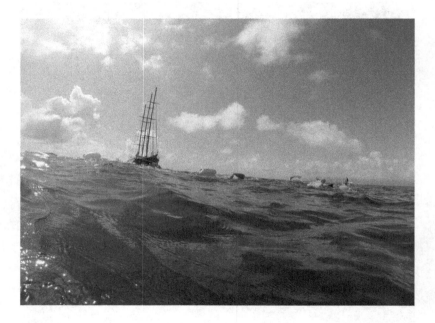

This is how we looked during a swimming training session: small dots in an enormous ocean.

When you realize, that you are in the middle of an ocean, with a depth of hundreds of meters, sometimes it can be frightening.

The diving was quite pleasant. We didn't see any manta rays

nor many sharks, but I always enjoy the calm atmosphere below the surface.

All in all, since learning to dive 15 months earlier, I have completed 17 dives in four countries: in Israel, in Maldives, in Costa Rica, and now in Seychelles.

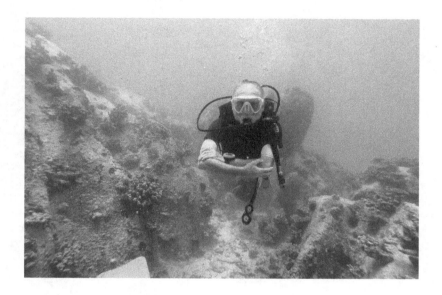

My swimming was OK. I wasn't exhausted after two hours, but except for the first session I used fins, so it wasn't a completely representative accomplishment.

But I enjoyed myself.

I would like to share with you two more photos of this beautiful place. Maybe it'll convince you to go there.

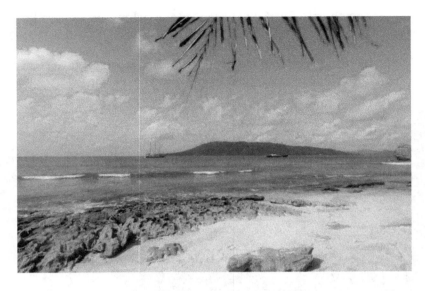

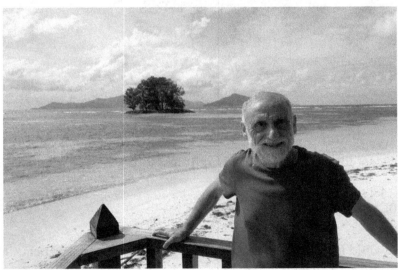

In summary: a challenging week, rough seas, a lot of swimming, some diving. Not sure I am swimming better now, but enjoyed it a lot.

CHAPTER 40
....
The Secrets of Success

During my diversified and quite successful career, I have faced many challenges and have succeeded in coping with them.

Now I am using this life experience to succeed in my sport activities.

I have tried to isolate and to analyze what were the ingredients of my success.

Here is a summary:
- The dream.
- The decision.
- The plan.
- The persistence.
- Visualizing.
- Not giving up.
- "The power within."

Everything begins with "the dream." If you don't dare to dream that you will achieve something, you obviously will not achieve it.

Then comes the decision: "I'm going to do it!"

To accomplish anything, you need a plan – begin planning: first a more general, high level plan, and then a detailed plan.

There will always be ups and downs; persistence is a key ingredient on the way to success.

Visualize the outcome. Try to see it happening. It will eventually become real.

It may be difficult – don't give up!

We all have a lot of inner power, hidden deep inside. We only need to reach-out, or rather reach-in, and get it!

Good luck!

CHAPTER 41
....
The Fourth Half-Marathon, Tel Aviv

After returning from Seychelles I give running the highest priority.

All my runs are faster than before. Maybe simply because I "push" a bit harder.

On Wednesday, January 29th, the date I was "reborn" twice, I ran a standard 8 kilometers. But after 4 kilometers, when I was at the most distant point of the track, it began to rain.

Initially it was a light "delicate" rain. But the last two kilometers were in a heavy rain.

I took it easy, if I were swimming I would also be wet.

When I got home I took a hot shower and felt perfect.

Rain isn't a reason for becoming ill.

I said that on January 29th I was "reborn" twice.

I see this date as my "additional" birthday; on January 29th 1969 I arrived in Israel, after leaving Poland – it was a key milestone in my life and a real "game changer."

On January 29th 2002 I was literally born again – receiving my life back. Following chemotherapy and radiotherapy I underwent surgery to remove my colorectal stage three (out of four) cancer.

At the time, my probability of survival was less than 30 percent, but the treatments and the surgery were successful and I survived.

All in all, in the short month of February I ran almost 100 kilometers.

My routine includes going to the fitness center three times a week. But there is one exercise I do at home, 2 to 3 times a week, which I believe contributes greatly to building up my core muscles, crucial to my performing well at any sport.

I mean the Plank.

Below is a short description.

The Plank Exercise: *Lie face down with legs extended and elbows bent and directly under shoulders; clasp your hands. Feet should be hip-width apart, and elbows should be shoulder-width apart. Contract your abs (abdominal muscles), then tuck your toes to lift your body (forearms remain on the ground); you should be in a straight line from head to heels. Hold or as long as you can.*

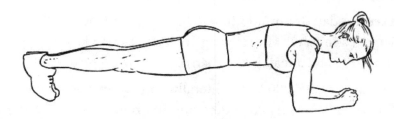

We began with 30 seconds, the next time 40, then 50 and after a few weeks I could hold the position for three minutes.

As with any exercise, progress requires staying at each level for some time. If you have sufficient patience, it can be up to a week at each level.

If you are a less patient person, then repeat each level 2 to 3 times and then progress to the next level.

If you want to flatten your stomach, the Plank is the perfect exercise.

I warmly recommend you trying it. Investing 2 to 3 minutes, three times a week, will result in effects out of proportion to the time invested.

Plank isn't an easy exercise. Until recently I was holding it for up to three minutes.

But this month I pushed myself to the limits, prolonging the time by 10 to 20 seconds every two days: 3:30, 4 minutes, 4:30, 5 minutes, 5:20, 5:40 and on February 9th 5:50!

Another thing I intend to change in my 4th half marathon is to give up the belt with the two small bottles, to rely on the water stations and to run more easily. I will carry only two gels, two dates, two electrolytes tablets and the keys to the car.

I also intend to run the last long run before – 15 kilometers, on Tuesday, February 11th – 17 days before the race.

After that only 5 to 7 km runs, and the last one on Monday the 24th, leaving myself a substantial time to rest before the 21.1kms on February 28th. The idea is to keep the stores of glycogen full and to develop the "hunger" to run.

On Tuesday I wake up early, but go to run only at 6:30 AM.

It is a very cold morning, 6 degrees Celsius (43F) and a strong wind, over 30km/h.

I take along a light jacket, with the intention of using it for the first three kilometers and then, when passing close to my car, leaving it and taking the water backpack instead.

This thought helps me to cope with my fear of the cold.

But when the time comes, I don't implement it and run in a t-shirt and running shorts.

It is very cold. My hands are frozen and my nose is like a running faucet.

Also, I have to stop three times to pee! Probably because of the cold.

The 15 kilometers take me one hour and fifty minutes, including all the breaks.

This means that even if I have to take breaks during the Tel Aviv half marathon, and assuming that the last 6 kilometers take no more than 40 minutes, in the worst case I'll finish in two and a half hours.

But of course, I'll do my best to improve my time at least a bit, still aiming at finishing in two hours.

Most important is to avoid any issues with my knee.

After the run I devote 15 minutes to stretching. The wind dries the sweat very fast and again I start to feel really cold.

Now the light jacket turns out to be very handy.

Thanks to proper movements and a long stretch, I manage to avoid any pain or stiffness in the leg muscles, and actually feel that I could keep on running.

That afternoon I find myself walking near the Marathon sport store and stop to say hello to the owner, Eliezer, who two years earlier convinced me to try the Altra running shoes and thus forever changed my running experience.

Eliezer is a marathon runner and a coach, who is now in his sixties.

It appears that he saw my running records on Facebook, and had some important comments.

According to his experience, since I am able to run 10 kilometers in 53 to 54 minutes, there is no reason that I should not be able run a half marathon in two hours or less.

Eliezer suggests that I push harder during my long training runs, at least the last 5 kilometers should be run much faster.

I believe that Eliezer is right. I can do better.

Actually, recently, I have been having similar thoughts - I have to leave my "comfort zone" of the 6:20min/km pace, and two hours and 15 minutes for the half marathon.

On the other hand, it's a kind of funny. It is not a question anymore of whether or not I can run the half marathon. This is already a fact. The only question now is how fast can I run it.

Isn't this great news?!

Despite my already having several pairs of Altra shoes, I couldn't withstand the temptation, and bought the new Altra Torin Plush running shoe, which is supposed to offer the best protection for my sensitive left foot. This will be my "Altra #17...".

With continuing improvements, one day they will invent shoes that run by themselves. ☺

At the same time, I continue my training routine, with the exception of swimming. Every year the swimming pool is closed in February for maintenance.

But I do a kind of a "dry swimming exercise"; according to the WEST Technique I extend my arm as much as possible, and then – a bit more! This allows for longer gliding.

To practice swimming faster, I do it in a "windmill motion" moving the other hand in parallel, immediately as the first hand begins the catch.

Will have to wait, to see whether this "dry swimming exercise," which I invented, will improve my swimming.

Also, less cycling outside, because of the many days of heavy rain.

So, I devote more time to the gym, reaching one and a half hour sessions and more biking on my indoor bike trainer – a new record – two full hours, although not fast.

I continue enjoying dancing, 25 lessons so far.

Recently we learned Bachata, which was quite challenging and Rumba-Bolero. Real fun!

On Friday, February 14th, two weeks before the Tel Aviv half marathon, I decide to push more during my weekly 5km intervals run.

The first two kilometers go really well – at a pace of 5:15min/km.

I think my RPE (rating of perceived exertion) was 17 (i.e. "very hard" on the Borg RPE scale, (between 6 and 20)).

But I don't give up.

I eventually finish 5.3 kilometers in 28 minutes, at an average pace of 5:18minutes/km, one of my fastest runs ever.

But the biggest surprise is my average heart rate – only 136bpm! My lowest ever!

Also, the maximum heart rate was relatively very low as well – 156bpm!

So, it felt very hard, but what happened? Nothing! I'm OK and feel very satisfied.

The conclusion; I shall indeed leave my "comfort zone" and push more!

Friday, February 28th – the day has come.

In two days, on Sunday, March 1st, I'll be 69 and today I'm going to run my 4th half marathon!

I wake up at 4 AM, drink my traditional green tea and by 5, I have left the house.

5:20 AM, I arrive at the parking lot, still plenty of empty spaces.

A 2 kilometer walk to the race grounds. It's another world…

I'm walking in the dark when I suddenly arrive at a different world. Over 40,000 runners will be gathering here soon.

First my physiological needs (a long line…) and it is already 6 AM.

At 6:15, I move to the appointed, fenced off starting area.

I throw aside the light jacked I had been wearing against the early morning cold. I leave it for those who may need it.

In a light run, we all move to the pre-start area. Makes for a good warm-up, and I take a good starting position.

Since recently I have been running a bit faster, especially at the beginning, I prefer to be in the front lines. Otherwise, I will have to waste time and energy trying to find an opening to pass between the slower runners.

This time the wait isn't that long and at 6:30 AM the half marathon begins.

I am full of energy, highly motivated to improve my personal record.

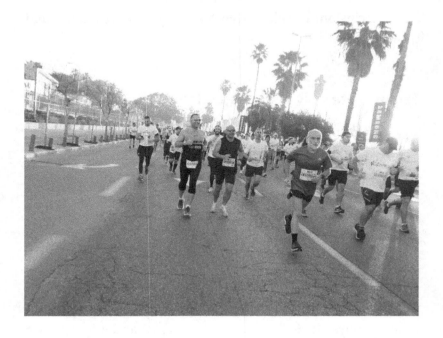

The first two kilometers go very well. Time: 11 minutes, at a pace of 5:30minutes/km.

I stumble on a pothole and almost fall. In a fraction of a second a thought passes through my mind – the race is over!

I stop to examine the damage. Fortunately, it isn't serious and I carefully resume running.

I finished the first 10 kilometers in one hour, still relatively well.

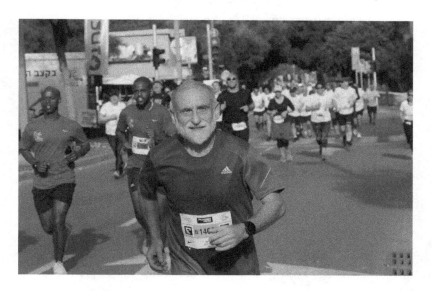

That morning, up until the last minute, I hesitated as to which shoes to wear: the well proven Altra Paradigm 4.5, with which I ran the first three half marathons, or the new Torin Plush, which I used in recent fast runs.

The Torin were also significantly lighter.

During the previous week I had by chance, run into Eliezer and he had strongly recommended that I use the Torin, which are better suited for a fast run, while still providing very good protection.

Eventually I followed Eliezer's advice and ran with the Torin.

But after the first 12 kilometers, the almost forgotten pain in my left forefoot once again returned, continuing to increase until finally reaching a level of 7 out of 10.

The pain also lasted for many long hours after the run.

Conclusion:

- Nobody knows my body, as well as I do.
- The next long run – Paradigm!

We run through slight climbs and descents and overall my pace starts to become a bit slower. Not a lot, but eventually my average pace turns out to be 6:14 minutes/km and I finish in two hours and eleven minutes.

A slight improvement of 4 minutes over the average of the first three half marathons.

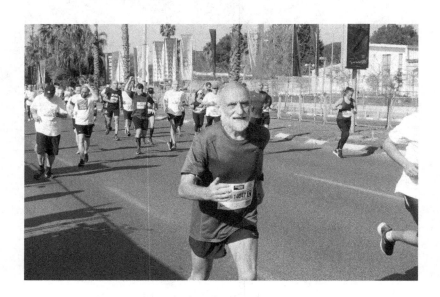

My RPE (rating of perceived exertion) was 15, or "Hard" according to the Borg RPE scale, but still OK.

Although my average heart rate was 162 bpm, exactly the lactic threshold, I was surprised to see, that my maximum heart rate had reached 192 bpm!

On the positive side, according to the formula MHR=220-age, it leads to the conclusion that I am only 28.

The following day, Saturday morning, I awoke at 4:30 AM and am happy to report that nothing was hurting!

It is less than 24 hours after the run, and it looks like I am fully recovered, no damage!

With satisfaction I can summarize this forth half marathon as follows: For the fourth time in four months I have run 21.1 kilometers, eventually achieving a slight improvement, enjoying it very much and am almost fully recovered in less than 24 hours.

But when I think about running a full marathon, the 42 kilometers, a year from now, it feels frightening...!

To summarize in one sentence: I loved the experience of my fourth half-marathon!

EPILOGUE
....

March 1st 2020. I'm 69 years old today, and a year from now I will run in the same place, my first full marathon.

But before that I have a full year of training and hard work. I intend to enjoy every moment, and especially the moments after.

I have achieved all of the goals that I set for myself for the 69th year of my life.

I feel good regarding my progress with the half marathon and it is now time to cross the Rubicon, and to move on toward the full marathon.

The story of this second stage will be told in the memoir that I am beginning today, and will conclude on my 70th birthday. So, I am stopping here.

Next week going on my traditional ski vacation and on the last day of March will run for the first time, 22 kilometers, as a first step toward running the marathon.

My plan for the coming year: extending the length of my runs by 1 kilometer each month, with the goal of reaching 32 kilometers by January 2021.

The remaining 10 kilometers will be a one-time, the biggest in my life effort, at the end of February 2021. I plan to release Part II of this memoir in April 2021, stay tuned. Wish me luck!

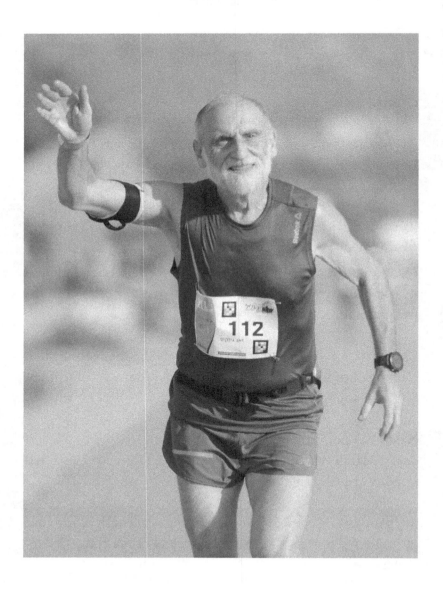

ABOUT THE AUTHOR
....

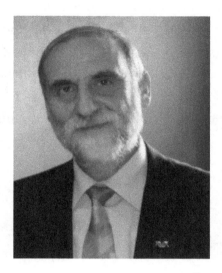

Zeev Gilkis, PhD, was the founder of AMIT, an institute for bio-medical development at Technion. For more than eight years he was the CEO of the institute and led the establishment of five start-ups in various fields of medicine, serving as the chairman of the Board of Directors of all five.

For over 11 years he held senior management positions at Comverse Technology which was at the time an S&P 500 company.

He earned his PhD with a thesis on Artificial Intelligence, and in addition, holds graduate degrees in mathematics, statistics and computer science and a Master of Science in mathematics.

Gilkis served in the mythological 8200 SIGINT unit of Israeli Intelligence for 17 years, and was awarded the highest "Award for Israeli National Security", by the President of Israel.

He served as the first Israeli military attaché to Poland and Hungary. In addition to his diversified career, he has devoted most of his free time to neuro-science, health and nutrition.

He is the author of the books: *Unlock Bliss, a Memoir of Getting Happier* and *The Secret of Life, a Memoir of Getting Younger.*

He is a vegan, and a practitioner of both yoga and meditation.

CPSIA information can be obtained
at www.ICGtesting.com
Printed in the USA
BVHW060306030920
587912BV00002B/187

9 789655 751598